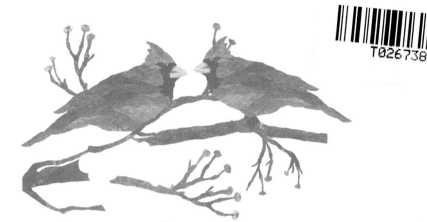

Cases and Concepts in
OCCUPATIONAL
ADAPTATION

Translating Theory into Action

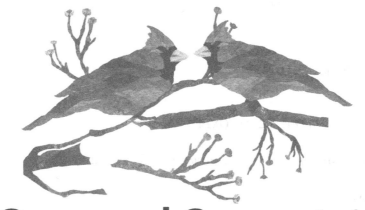

Cases and Concepts in
OCCUPATIONAL ADAPTATION

Translating Theory into Action

CYNTHIA LEE EVETTS, PhD, OTR, FAOTA

Professor and Director
School of Occupational Therapy
Texas Woman's University
Denton, Dallas, and Houston, Texas

MARY FRANCES BAXTER, PhD, OT, FAOTA

Professor and Associate Director
School of Occupational Therapy
Texas Woman's University
Houston, Texas

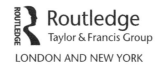

Routledge
Taylor & Francis Group

LONDON AND NEW YORK

Designed cover image: Tinhouse Design

First published 2024
by Routledge
605 Third Avenue, New York, NY 10017

and by Routledge
4 Park Square, Milton Park, Abingdon, Oxon, OX14 4RN

Routledge is an imprint of the Taylor & Francis Group, an informa business

ISBN: 9781630919689 (pbk)
ISBN: 9781003522850 (ebk)

DOI: 10.4324/9781003522850

Typeset in Minion Pro
by SLACK Incorporated

Dedication

This book is dedicated to practitioners and scholars who have shaped occupational adaptation theory over the past 3 decades. They used the power of occupation to enhance adaptive capacity, and thereby, participation in everyday living. We thank them for sharing their experiences.

We also acknowledge that adaptive capacity does not have to emerge under the supervision of a practitioner. We dedicate our labor to the memories of our mothers—strong women who encouraged us to aim high and strive to leave a place better than we found it. We hope to model how adaptive repertoire keeps us putting one foot in front of the other.

Contents

Acknowledgments

This scholarly work did not occur without the generous contributions of our students and colleagues. Each contributor of a story, case, or practice model is recognized by name; these contributions give life and breath to the theoretical concepts that might otherwise leave the reader muddled in their understanding. We are deeply appreciative to each and every one.

We thank the artists who provided graphics to illustrate some of the stories. We are grateful for their gift of time and talent and proud because they are our sons, Mitchell Reid and David Baxter, who actually get what we do.

We also recognize the additional contribution of editorial work by Brooke King who helped ensure the readable nature of the text and edited cases and stories to hone their focus in just-right ways.

About the Authors

Cynthia Lee Evetts, PhD, OTR, FAOTA is a professor and director of the School of Occupational Therapy at Texas Woman's University in Denton, Texas. Her educational background in industrial arts education, occupational therapy, and community health education fuels her desire to demonstrate the power of meaningful occupation to prompt adaptive behavior, enhance quality of life, and improve health.

Dr. Evetts was mentored by Drs. Janette K. Schkade and Sally Schultz who entertained her questions about occupational adaptation with enthusiasm, even when they did not completely agree in their answers. She now teaches the PhD course on occupational adaptation at Texas Woman's University and is energized and fascinated by how students consistently challenge her to join them in thinking deeply to explore theoretical constructs and ideas. She offers this shoutout to Jenny, Kyle, and Amber to keep up the "theory query," which started as a classroom blog and continues through conversations over Zoom.

Mary Frances Baxter, PhD, OT, FAOTA received her BS in occupational therapy from Colorado State University in Fort Collins, Colorado; her MA in rehabilitation technology for occcupational therapy from Texas Woman's University in Denton, Texas; and her PhD in kinesiology and health from the University of Houston in Houston, Texas. She is currently a professor in the School of Occupational Therapy at Texas Woman's University and serves as the associate director of the Houston campus.

Dr. Baxter identifies as a generalist occupational therapy practitioner and has a strong background in neuroscience for occupational therapy, as well as a range of clinical practice areas, including pediatrics, physical disabilities, oncology, and assistive technology. She has been an academic faculty member for more than 30 years, teaching students across all levels of education, including the PhD program.

Dr. Baxter's focused areas of scholarship include occupational therapy in oncology care and survivorship, creativity with support from neuroscience in occupational therapy, and the effects of postural control on participation. She has a record of publications in all her areas of research, including eight book chapters and numerous published articles, and presents regularly at state, national, and international conferences.

About Our Colleagues

Janette K. Schkade, after graduating with a PhD in psychology, practiced as a psychologist in a state school for persons with intellectual disabilities, working with clients who had multiple physical, as well as mental, disabilities. It was in this environment that she learned about occupational therapy and what it could do for this population. She then obtained her education in occupational therapy from Texas Woman's University in Denton, Texas. She is a coauthor of the occupational adaptation theoretical framework. She presented at national and regional conferences on this framework, both as theory and as a vehicle to guide practice. She is the author or coauthor of numerous publications regarding occupational adaptation, both in scholarly journals and book chapters.

Dr. Schkade retired in 2001, moved to an idyllic home in the beautiful mountains of Arkansas, and left this world a better place when she died in 2008. We miss her leadership and vision, her playful spirit, and her enthusiasm for life.

Melissa McClung had been practicing with the occupational adaptation theoretical perspective for 10 years. She had the opportunity to use the theory in practice with patients, in redesigning existing occupational therapy programs, in student programs in clinic settings, and in classroom curriculum design/implementation as a faculty member at Texas Woman's University. She had presented her approach to occupational adaptation at national and regional conferences. Prior to becoming an occupational therapist, she practiced as a music therapist for 8 years.

McClung died far too soon in 2009, cutting short a successful career in occupational therapy and leaving behind her children, Bailey and Teague. We miss her laughter and singing in the halls, her strong connection with students, and her dedication to the profession.

The red birds on the cover of this book are in reference to the saying, "When red birds appear a loved one is near." Dr. Schkade and McClung are gone from this earth but not forgotten in our hearts and minds and are reflected in this volume, which was based on the framework they laid out in *Occupational Adaptation in Practice: Concepts and Cases* (2001, SLACK Incorporated).

Contributors

Alondra Ammon, MOT, OTR/L (Chapters 2 and 6)
Adjunct Instructor and Occupational Therapist
Department of Occupational Therapy
Samuel Merritt University
Oakland, California

Lindsay Ballew, MOT, OTR/L (Chapter 3)
Texas Woman's University
Denton, Texas

Gail Blom, OTR, CHT, CLT, MA (Chapter 4)
Owner and Therapist
Covenant Hand Therapy, PC
Plano, Texas

Jessica Dolecheck, PhD, OTR (Retired) (Chapter 4)
Professor and Program Director
Health Studies Department
College of Health Sciences
University of Louisiana Monroe
Monroe, Louisiana

Christine E. Haines, PhD, OTR
(Chapters 7 and 12)
Occupational Therapist
Physical Medicine and Rehabilitation
Michael E. DeBakey Veterans Affairs Medical Center
Houston, Texas

DeLana Honaker, PhD, OTR (Chapter 4)
Deceased

Catherine Evich Johnson, OTS (Chapter 10)

Jessica Johnson, OTR, MOT (Chapter 12)
Owner and Lead Occupational Therapy Practitioner
Thrive n Play
Lewisville, Texas

Kristin Bray Jones, MS, OTD, OTR/L (Chapter 1)
Assistant Professor and Academic Fieldwork Coordinator
Occupational Therapy Department
Dominican University of California
San Rafael, California

Kyle Karen, MS, PhD (Chapters 2 and 4)
Assistant Professor
Department of Occupational Therapy
New York Institute of Technology
Old Westbury, New York

Brooke King, MSOT, OTR/L (Chapters 3, 9, 10, and 12)
PhD Candidate
School of Occupational Therapy
Texas Woman's University
Houston, Texas

Joanna Lipoma, MOT, OTR (Chapters 4 and 10)

Christene Maas, PhD, MA, OTR (Chapter 12)
Assistant Professor
Department of Occupational Therapy
University of the Incarnate Word
San Antonio, Texas

Melissa McClung, MOT, OTR (Chapter 6)
Deceased

Kimberly Norton, MA, LOTR, CHT (Chapter 4)

Emily M. Rich, MOT, OTR/L (Chapter 5)
Occupational Therapist
Outpatient Therapies
Tucson Medical Center
Tucson, Arizona

Stefanie Casey Rogers, PhD, OTR (Chapter 3)
Occupational Therapist
Children's Health Rehabilitation and Therapy Services
Children's Health–Children's Medical Center
Dallas, Texas

Teri K. Rupp, PhD, OTR/L, C/NDT (Chapter 5)
Pediatric Occupational Therapist
Auburn School District 408
Auburn, Washington

Sarah Rupp-Blanchard, OTD, MHA, OTR (Chapter 6)
President and Administrator
Milestone Therapy Services
Dallas, Texas

Michelle S. Scheffler, OTR, MOT (Chapter 13)
Occupational Therapist
Houston, Texas

Stephanie Springfield, OTS (Chapter 2)

Anne Sullivan, PhD, OTR (Chapter 6)
Assistant Professor
School of Occupational Therapy
Texas Woman's University
Dallas, Texas

Savitha Sundar, MS, OTR/L (Chapter 13)
Partnerships Officer
Changing Perspectives
Sacramento, California
Montpelier, Vermont

Nanette Tabani, OTS (Chapter 2)

Orley A. Templeton, MS, OTD, OTR/L, CAS (Chapter 8)
Assistant Professor
Occupational Therapy Department
Misericordia University
Dallas, Pennsylvania

Jennifer K. Whittaker, MSOT, OTR/L, CPH, CHES (Chapter 10)
Adjunct Faculty
Department of Occupational Therapy
Department of Health and Human Performance
The University of Scranton
Scranton, Pennsylvania
PhD Candidate
School of Occupational Therapy
Texas Woman's University
Denton, Texas

Preface

This book follows a 2001 publication introducing the then-budding theory in *Occupational Adaptation in Practice: Concepts and Cases* by our dearly departed colleagues and friends Dr. Janette K. Schkade and Melissa McClung. Their early work and desire to make occupational adaptation theory accessible to students and practitioners inspired our efforts to update the language, include the research that informs occupational adaptation theory, and provide fresh examples of cases and practice models that exemplify its application.

Dr. Schkade and McClung believed "that theory is extremely useful in guiding a practice that is versatile, effective, and efficient. However, the usefulness of theory depends on the therapist having a working understanding of the principles. A thorough understanding enables the therapist to be creative and responsive to the dynamic needs of the client" (Schkade & McClung, 2001).

Developed as part of a planning process for the PhD in occupational therapy program at Texas Woman's University in Denton, Texas, occupational adaptation was designed to provide a research focus and to be a guide for therapeutic intervention. Occupational adaptation first appeared in print in a two-part article in the *American Journal of Occupational Therapy* (Schkade & Schultz, 1992; Schultz & Schkade, 1992).

Here is what you can expect as you read this book: Each chapter starts with a quote that enhances the theme to follow. We have linked concepts and constructs from professional literature that illustrate how studies related to occupational adaptation have contributed to our understanding. We have included several references to Eleanor Clarke Slagle lectures that align with the theory and its application in order to show congruence with renowned thinkers and trends in occupational therapy. Fresh and varied cases have been added to further illustrate what it looks like to apply theory in practice. The neuroscience that underlies the occupational adaptation process is explained to help the reader connect both the art and the science of occupational therapy. Worksheets are provided to prompt application to self and also to practice applying theory to client-centered scenarios. We think this text will be useful to the novice, as well as the seasoned, practitioner, for whom we have included "A Deeper Dive" to challenge application even further into practice and occupational science. Finally, we end by sharing occupational adaptation practice models designed by occupational therapists to guide both traditional and innovative practice.

We agree with Dr. Schkade and McClung's intent and we also "hope that this book will increase your commitment to, your enjoyment of, and your excitement about the practice of client-centered occupational therapy" (Schkade & McClung, 2001).

—*Cynthia Lee Evetts, PhD, OTR, FAOTA and Mary Frances Baxter, PhD, OT, FAOTA*

References

Schkade, J. K., & McClung, M. (2001). *Occupational adaptation in practice: Concepts and cases*. SLACK Incorporated.

Schkade, J. K., & Schultz, S. (1992). Occupational adaptation: Toward a holistic approach to contemporary practice, part 1. *American Journal of Occupational Therapy, 46,* 829-837.

Schultz, S., & Schkade, J. K. (1992). Occupational adaptation: Toward a holistic approach to contemporary practice, part 2. *American Journal of Occupational Therapy, 46,* 917-926.

Before You Begin

A Few Words About the Theory of Occupational Adaptation

- Occupational adaptation describes a "normal" process. Everybody has the need and opportunity to adapt all the time. Therefore, you may see yourself and be able to reflect on your own experiences as you come to understand how the theory explains a very normal process.
- The adaptive process is easily disrupted, especially during periods of transition or stress. Disrupted adaptation can lead to dysfunction.
- Restoration of the adaptive process is the focus of intervention from an occupational adaptation perspective. Skill acquisition is not the focus.
- The client's capacity to engage in preferred life roles is the ultimate goal.

A Few Words About How This Book Is Designed to Promote Understanding of the Theory of Occupational Adaptation

- Each chapter focuses on how a particular occupational adaptation concept contributes to both function and dysfunction.
- Real cases contributed by practicing therapists are strategically placed in the book as examples of occupational adaptation concepts in practice.
- A "Try It On" feature in most chapters enhances understanding through personal application. This feature has been designed to have the reader apply occupational adaptation to a personal situation. The reader will use the same personal situation throughout the book.

CHAPTER 1

Overview of the Occupational Adaptation Theory
What's Occupational Adaptation?

*Occupational adaptation is a way to name
and frame what good therapists do.*
—Janette K. Schkade

Occupational adaptation is (a) a concept that describes a human phenomenon, (b) a framework that therapists can use to guide their intervention planning and implementation, and c) a theory used to predict adaptive response outcomes. The construct of occupational adaptation described in this book emerged from deep conversations about what makes good occupational therapy. These conversations were held among faculty members at Texas Woman's University as they worked to develop a PhD program in occupational therapy in the early 1990s. The construct evolved by describing how enduring concepts in occupational therapy come together to explain good occupational therapy and what good occupational therapists do to facilitate positive outcomes.

Occupational adaptation as it was first articulated is one description of a process thought to be present in all human beings (Schkade & Schultz, 1992; Schultz & Schkade, 1992). This process exists in humans to allow us to respond masterfully and adaptively to the various occupational challenges that we encounter over a lifetime. The adaptation process is supported by concepts in neuroscience in that cellular and neural systems exhibit some form of adaptation, which provides the ability to constantly detect and respond to changes in the person or environment. We believe that this process provides the tools that humans need to develop and sustain competence in carrying out the tasks associated with the various life roles we take on (i.e., competence in occupational functioning).

Evetts, C. L., & Baxter, M. F. *Cases and Concepts in Occupational Adaptation: Translating Theory into Action* (pp. 1-6). DOI: 10.4324/9781003522850-1

Life roles provide the context for expressing our competence in occupational functioning. The occupational adaptation process is a strengths-based approach for carrying out these roles adaptively and masterfully. The tasks contained in life roles change from time to time, requiring us to adapt to be successful. We also believe that demand on the occupational adaptation process is greatest when the individual must transition to changing life roles. The importance of transition to occupational therapy practitioners was emphasized by Dr. Karen Jacobs during her 2012 Eleanor Clarke Slagle lecture as follows: "People decompensate when they are undergoing transitions; … this is an important factor for occupational therapy practitioners to be aware of because we almost always see people in the midst of a transition in their lives" (Jacobs, 2012, p. 655). The greater the transition, the higher the risk the occupational adaptation process is disrupted. For example, a person with an acute spinal cord injury faces major life transitions in areas of occupational functioning, such as work, leisure, and self-care. Even if that person's occupational adaptation process is functioning adequately, it is likely to become dysfunctional under such an extreme challenge.

Before we examine a clinical case, let us look at a common experience that does not involve an injury, illness, or disabling condition. The story of The New Mom (Story 1-1) offers one example of how the need for individuals to adapt in ordinary life circumstances can appear. We illustrate this normative process through the transition of Jill to the role of a first-time mother.

Jill's challenging day can be described in terms of the occupational adaptation process. Jill had the skills necessary to check off each task on her list, but despite her capability, she was unsuccessful. This is the primary difference between occupational adaptation and other occupation-based theories; although others assume that if a person has occupational performance skills, then they will be successful in occupational participation, occupational adaptation assumes that if a person is adaptive, then they will both participate and perform with relative mastery (Cole, 2011; Schultz, 2009).

If, as we suggest, the occupational adaptation process is the means by which we develop and sustain competence in occupational functioning, then it seems logical that a healthy process is most likely to result in meeting the challenges. The occupational adaptation process facilitates the development of life skills that must be adapted to any change in a person's capabilities. Therefore, the repair or restoration of the occupational adaptation process is critical. Thus, the therapist who practices from an occupational adaptation perspective intervenes from the assumption that the therapeutic task is to facilitate a healthy occupational adaptation process in the client. This point of view empowers the client to be their own agent of competence development. The therapist simply but skillfully and very importantly sets the stage for this process to unfold and function at its best. In Case 1-1, traditional rehabilitation alone is unable to help Connie move past her pain and loss of function.

It is important to recognize that the occupational adaptation process is a "normative" process. This means that it is not just something that operates in people who have experienced disease, trauma, or stress. It operates in everyone regardless of health status. At one time or another, each of us has been occupationally dysfunctional. Some of us have been so more frequently or for longer periods of time than others have been, but we have all experienced dysfunction. Therefore, we recommend that a therapist wishing to use this perspective in intervention should first "try it on" in their own life role adaptation challenges. If it seems to "fit," then the therapist

---

STORY 1-1

The New Mom

Jill is a physically active person who is organized and thoughtful. She generally plans well, thinks things through, and enjoys making lists for her day's tasks. She worked in a fast-paced industry up until the birth of her child. Now, Jill is elated with motherhood, choosing to be a stay-at-home mom while her husband, Jack, is the primary breadwinner for the family. As Jill entered motherhood, she desired a loved, well-cared-for baby while keeping an organized home, adapting to the growing family's needs. On this day, Jill's to-do list includes taking care of and spending quality time with her baby, tidying the living space, providing a nutritious meal for herself and Jack, and running errands. Jill notes she had offered to pick up their dry cleaning, which will help Jack because he has a business meeting tomorrow and a clean suit would be nice. Jill starts off the day with focus, direction, and exuberant amounts of energy; however, her plans are interrupted by an unexpected visitor, a playdate that goes into overtime and car trouble while running errands. Thus, by evening, Jack arrives home to find Jill frustrated by the day's events and her lack of success in completing her to-do list. Jill makes a mental note to repeat the same plan tomorrow and to try harder.

Jill's decision to try the same plan again although it did not work the first time reflects how, in normal life transitions, we may fail to adapt even when there is a need for adaptation. Jill may wind up repeating this dysfunctional pattern more than once before she perceives any need for adaptation. Jill's occupational adaptation process will have to be more functional if she is to experience success in her new role.

CASE 1-1

The Knitter

Connie was 50 years old and worked as a night shift stocker for a discount department store. I saw Connie in an outpatient rehabilitation clinic for a wrist sprain she sustained after carrying heavy boxes of clothing. She was off work because of this disability and mentioned how much she wanted to get back to work.

In learning more about Connie, it seemed that her job was one of few occupations she engaged in. She lived with her mother and slept most of the day and then went to work at night. She would spend any free time watching television with her mom. In general, Connie had a flat affect and seemed shy or uncomfortable when talking to me. I noted she did not look at or talk to anyone else in the open clinic area.

It was surprising to me that her clinical progress was slow given her desire to go back to work and compliance with the home exercise program. Given the slowness of her progress, I gave her case a second look. I acknowledged that the current treatment plan was not going to meet Connie's goal of returning to work. I reflected on Connie's flat affect and shyness. I reflected on the limited roles that Connie mentioned in our conversations.

At our next session, I moved Connie to a more private area of the clinic and asked about her interest and experience with crafts. She said she did not have much experience but was willing to learn. That session, I taught Connie the beginning steps for knitting. The goals for therapy continued to be the same (i.e., to increase range of motion, strength, and activity tolerance and to decrease pain) but what quickly emerged was Connie's identification with a new role—a knitter, maker, and crafter.

Soon after Connie began knitting, I observed a dramatic shift in Connie's pain and affect. Her pain decreased, and she seemed more comfortable engaging with me and others in the clinic. Eventually, as her wrist improved, she would ask to stay past her 30-minute appointment time so she could knit a bit more. Connie's range of motion, strength, and activity tolerance also improved. In fact, it was hard to keep her from only doing a therapeutic amount of knitting. Eventually, she took the knitting home with her and came back to show us a scarf she had made.

Connie provides an example of the power that a person's role has on their engagement in occupation. By adjusting an ineffective treatment plan to incorporate meaningful activities with new demands and a just-right challenge, Connie was given the opportunity to explore and identify with a new role. The result was that Connie's injury improved, and she shifted from a treatment receiver to someone actively engaged in the rehabilitation process. The holistic gains that were not measured but that were of equal importance were Connie's increased comfort with social interaction and clearly observable confidence in her new skills.

Case contributed by Kristin Bray Jones, MS, OTD, OTR/L

will better understand the practical application of the theory and adaptation process, and thus, be more equipped to use it as a guide to intervention. If it does not seem to have some kind of practical validity, using it in practice with a sufficient understanding to intervene effectively may be more difficult.

Figure 1-1 depicts a cross section of the occupational adaptation process, artificially stopped in time for us to examine the concepts and their relationships more closely. This "freeze-frame" approach depicts a stationary image of the process, much as one sees a computed tomographic scan cross-section of the brain or spine. You can see the structures and note some relationships regarding proximity and appearance; however, the image on the scan does not convey the dynamic nature of the ways in which these structures interact in routine functioning. The same thing is true of the occupational adaptation process figure. In real time, the process may be proceeding rapidly, and the individual will likely be dealing with multiple challenges at the same time or in quick succession. Our

discussions in the subsequent chapters also "stop" the process so that you can examine it more closely and thereby gain a deeper understanding of the concepts, their relationships, and the flow of the process. This does not imply a linear process.

The purpose of this book is to facilitate understanding of the occupational adaptation process and to make it therapeutically useful. Chapters are organized around the components of the process as seen in Figure 1-1. Explanations of each component include case examples contributed by therapists who have used this framework in practice. We also provide worksheets and answer keys to help you think through the application of the theory to actual practice.

There are important principles of intervention to keep in mind as you read the chapters. These principles are provided in Table 1-1. If you do not understand the terms at first glance, do not worry. The remaining chapters and case descriptions will bring them to life through skillful application by therapists with actual clients.

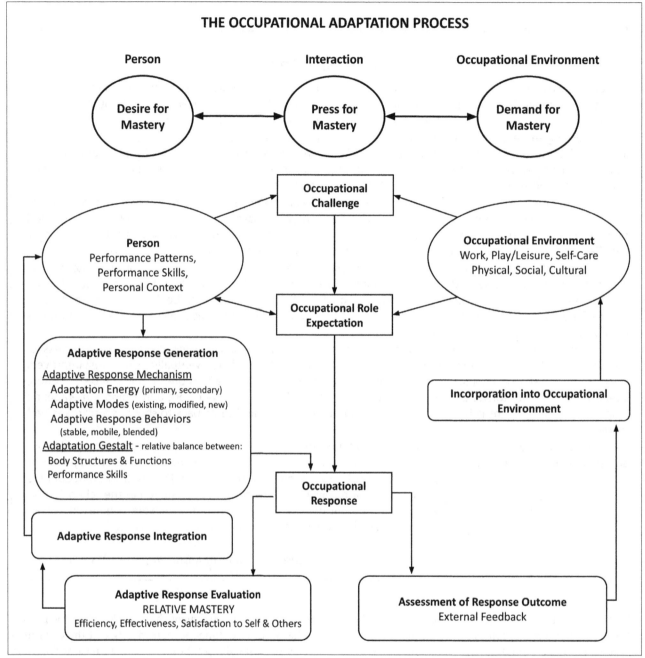

Figure 1-1. The occupational adaptation process. (Adapted from Schkade, J., & Schultz, S. [1992]. Occupational adaptation: Toward a holistic approach for contemporary practice, part 1. *American Journal of Occupational Therapy, 46*, 829-837.)

A therapist intervening with occupational adaptation must remember the following three "essentials" as the therapeutic process unfolds:

1. Your client will more likely achieve their goals if the internal adaptation process is working well. As with any intervention plan, revisions may be necessary if the adaptation process is not responding well to the plan and client goals are not being met.

2. There are three constant factors present in this process:

   a. The person desires to function masterfully and adaptively.

   b. The occupational environment demands mastery of the person.

   c. The interaction of the desire for mastery and the demand for mastery produces the press for mastery in the form of an occupational challenge. If your client does not demonstrate this desire, you cannot assume that it is absent in the client. Your conclusion should be that you have not identified the occupational role and goal that will allow this desire to be demonstrated. Therefore, you must continue to seek a client-relevant goal in consultation and collaboration with the client and/or family as illustrated in Case 1-1.

TABLE 1-1

Guiding Principles for Intervention

1. Occupational adaptation is a way of directing the therapist's thinking about intervention in an individual's internal adaptation process, not a collection of techniques.

2. Intervention is guided by meaningful, client-identified requirements of an occupational role, not by concerns about skill development. This role takes place within an environmental context about which the client or family must educate the therapist. Evaluation of strengths and deficits in Client Factors and Performance Skills[a] is measured against what promotes or inhibits the client's ability to carry out the meaningful role.

3. A personally meaningful intervention focused on the internal adaptation process will be more efficient and the outcomes more likely to generalize to other contexts than intervention focused on general skill development.

4. Intervention is characterized by a combination of methods.
   a. Occupational readiness addresses deficits in the Body Functions and Structure.[a] These interventions prepare (or "ready") systems to engage in occupation.
   b. Occupational activities simulate or replicate tasks of the meaningful occupational role, which guides intervention and directs the focus on the client's internal adaptation process. These activities must meet the three required properties for occupations: active participation by the client, meaning to the client, and process ending in a tangible or intangible product.

5. The client evaluates their progress in terms of relative mastery.
   a. Use of time, energy, and resources (efficiency)
   b. Extent to which the desired goal was achieved (effectiveness)
   c. Degree to which the personal actions producing the outcome were personally and socially well regarded (satisfaction to self and relevant to others)

6. The therapist assesses client progress with standard assessment tools and with indications that the client's internal adaptation process has been affected, including the following:
   a. Spontaneous generalization to other activities
   b. Initiation of new approaches in novel situations
   c. Increase in relative mastery

[a]Language updated to align with American Occupational Therapy Association. (2020). *Occupational therapy practice framework: Domain and process* (4th ed.). Author.

Adapted with permission from Schultz, S., & Schkade, J. (1997). Adaptation. In C. Christiansen & C. Baum (Eds.), *Occupational therapy: Enabling function and well-being* (2nd ed., p. 476). SLACK Incorporated.

---

3. Occupational adaptation intervention requires a holistic perspective of the client, and the whole person is inevitably present in every occupational response. This is true regardless of the setting in which you practice. Clients who struggle to function with cognitive or psychological problems are not exempt from physical impairment, and clients with musculoskeletal deficits are not immune from neurologic disorders or emotional responses to occupational challenges.

The plan for this book is to lead you through the process and use actual case studies to illustrate the use of occupational adaptation in practice. As each concept is introduced, a case is offered that emphasizes that particular concept. As you progress, you will recognize many concepts other than the one that is featured; this is because all concepts are present in every case. However, we use this approach to facilitate understanding of the major concepts and how they can be used in practice.

We do not attempt to tell you precisely what to "do" as an intervention. Occupational adaptation is a way of thinking about intervention from a client-centered, occupation-focused perspective. The Occupational Adaptation Guide to Practice, which is presented in Chapter 9 (adapted from Schultz & Schkade, 1992), is a series of questions, not a list of prescriptions. This guide offers questions to ask when practicing from an occupational adaptation perspective and guides your professional reasoning process. The answers to these questions shape your interaction with the client because together you develop a plan for occupational intervention. Additional guidelines for intervention are provided in Chapters 9 and 10.

We hope that you will find this book to be a useful tool for intervention that we believe will maximize the contributions of both the client and the therapist to a satisfying outcome that is client centered and occupationally focused.

References

Cole, M. B. (2011). *Group dynamics in occupational therapy: The theoretical basis and practice application of group intervention* (4th ed., pp. 291-294). SLACK Incorporated.

Jacobs, K. (2012). PromOTing occupational therapy: Words, images, and actions (Eleanor Clarke Slagle lecture). *American Journal of Occupational Therapy, 66,* 652-671. https://doi.org/10.5014/ajot.2012.666001

Schkade, J. K., & Schultz, S. (1992). Occupational adaptation: Toward a holistic approach to contemporary practice, part 1. *American Journal of Occupational Therapy, 46,* 829-837.

Schultz, S., & Schkade, J. K. (1992). Occupational adaptation: Toward a holistic approach to contemporary practice, part 2. *American Journal of Occupational Therapy, 46,* 917-926.

Schultz, S. (2009). Theory of occupational adaptation. In E. B. Crepeau, E. S. Cohn, & B. A. B. Schell (Eds.), *Willard & Spackman's occupational therapy* (11th ed., pp. 462-475). Lippincott Williams & Wilkins.

CHAPTER 2

Desire for Mastery, Demand for Mastery, Press for Mastery

How Do the Person and the Environment Relate?

Early Bird
Oh, if you're a bird, be an early bird
And catch the worm for your breakfast plate.
If you're a bird, be an early bird—
But if you're a worm, sleep late.
—*Shel Silverstein (2014, p. 30)*

As illustrated in Figure 1-1, two basic premises of occupational adaptation are (a) an individual desires to behave masterfully, and (b) the environment demands mastery of the person. The interaction between these two aspects results in a press for mastery in the form of an occupational challenge. As Dr. Ellen Cohn emphasized in her Eleanor Clarke Slagle lecture, "environments are not just containers for occupations; rather, our engagement in occupations is always situated, supported, and restricted by the physical, sociocultural, economic, temporal, technological, institutional, and political environments" (2019, p. 3). This chapter explores the multifaceted ways that mastery takes shape in the occupational adaptation process.

The desire for mastery, the demand for mastery, and the press for mastery are present throughout life. The desire and demand for mastery produce a dynamic tension between the individual, who desires to confront challenges adaptively and masterfully, and the environment, which demands that the individual respond adaptively and masterfully. Shel Silverstein's poem "Early Bird" (2014) presented at the opening of this chapter is a humorous illustration of how one environment interacts differently with two individuals. In this example, the bird demonstrates its desire for mastery over obtaining breakfast by waking early to get first dibs on any eatables, whereas the worm would desire not to be eaten and therefore stay hidden while the bird is still hungry. Each of the players in this scenario (both the bird and the worm) are

Evetts, C. L., & Baxter, M. F. *Cases and Concepts in Occupational Adaptation:*
Translating Theory into Action (pp. 7-15).
DOI: 10.4324/9781003522850-2

at once representing their own person systems while simultaneously playing a role in the environment of the other. At times, individuals shape an interaction that is adaptive and masterful. At other times, they do not. Competence in the interaction between an individual and their environment is a function of the health and strength of the occupational adaptation process as it develops over time, beginning with birth. Competence can be viewed as relative influence over the outcomes of a person–environment interaction.

Development of Mastery

The desire for mastery exists in a rudimentary form at birth. As the infant experiences some degree of perceived mastery (which emerges serendipitously from random and reflexive action), a repertoire of adaptive occupational responses begins to accumulate, and the occupational adaptation process starts to develop. The development of desire for mastery begins with the fundamental need for nutrition because the infant is challenged with locating the nipple at feeding time. At first reflexive, the nutrition-seeking approach adapts over time toward intentional behavior.

NEURO SPOTLIGHT

Neuroplasticity

In the neuroscience literature, adaptation occurs because of an attribute known as *neuroplasticity*. A broad definition of neuroplasticity is the ability of the neurons and the nervous system to reorganize structure, function, and connections in response to intrinsic and extrinsic stimuli. Neuroplasticity occurs at all levels across the nervous system, including molecular systems, cellular structures and processes, and in the changes in behavioral levels of function. The processes of neuroplasticity occur throughout the life span and are critical to development. Additional changes in neural structures and processes may occur as part of a disease process, as a response to environmental factors, or because of therapy. Engaging in activity naturally leads to changes in neural structures and processes as a person learns and encodes memories. Neuroplasticity plays a critical role in development, learning, memory, body functions, and behaviors that occupational therapists observe and measure.

How does the environment help elicit neuroplastic changes? Stimuli in the environment produce changes in the nervous system as the result of three basic processes: potentiation, habituation, and sensitization. Potentiation is the strengthening of a nerve synapse and is best described by the phrase "cells that fire together, wire together." Long-term potentiation is considered a major cellular mechanism that contributes to learning and memory. Habituation is the process of decreasing responses to repeated environmental stimuli (Figure 2-1). In habituation, fewer presynaptic neurotransmitters are released at the synapse, thus decreasing the response of the neuron. Habituation is at play when you adjust to wearing a new watch; at first you notice the heaviness of the watch on your wrist, and over time you forget you are wearing it. Conversely, in sensitization, more presynaptic neurotransmitters are released; therefore, the neuron is more excitable. Sensitization to a stimulus is the process in which there is an increased reaction to a paired second stimulus. It is often a startle response that is exaggerated and is frequently observed in trauma survivors. In these ways, neuroplasticity is a central component of occupational adaptation.

RECOMMENDED READINGS

Cohen, L. G., Celnik, P., Pascual-Leone, A., Corwell, B., Falz, L., Dambrosia, J., Honda, M., Sadato, N., Gerloff, C., Catala, M. D., & Hallett, M. (1997). Functional relevance of cross-modal plasticity in blind humans. *Nature, 389*(6647), 180-183. https://doi.org/10.1038/38278

Cramer, S. C., Sur, M., Dobkin, B. H., O'Brien, C., Sanger, T. D., Trojanowski, J. Q., Rumsey, J. M., Hicks, R., Cameron, J., Chen, D., Chen, W. G., Cohen, L. G., deCharms, C., Duffy, C. J., Eden, G. F., Fetz, E. E., Filart, R., Freund, M., Grant, S. J., ... Vinogradov, S. (2011). Harnessing neuroplasticity for clinical applications. *Brain, 134*(6), 1591-1609. https://doi.org/10.1093/brain/awr039

Puderbaugh, M., & Emmady, P. D. (2021). *Neuroplasticity*. StatPearls Publishing.

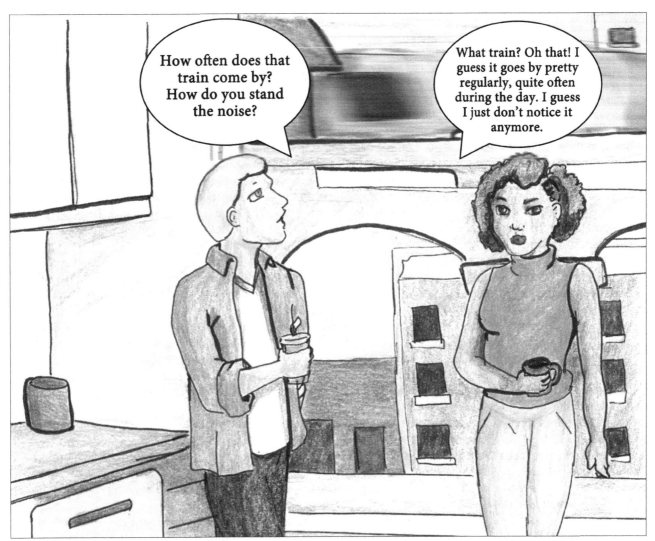

Figure 2-1. In her apartment near the tracks, Sophie has habituated to the noise of the commuter train that is quite obvious to visitors. (Illustrated by David Baxter.)

Toddlers demonstrate the desire for mastery during play. Toddlers demonstrate goal-directed behaviors by reaching for objects, gathering toys closer to the body, and producing some change in the object, such as separation, noise production, or shape manipulation. Adaptations of posture, movement, effort, and focus can be seen as the toddler attempts to achieve goals. The desire to master these challenges is obvious even to the casual observer as the toddler seeks to express influence over the environment.

Environmental characteristics shape the demand for mastery as both facilitators and barriers. For example, consider a child placed in a playpen. The physical barrier of the playpen shapes performance by constraining the toddler's explorations within the parameters of that space. A child placed on the floor is free to explore wider boundaries of the room. Social and cultural elements of the environment further influence the demand for mastery. Differences in child-rearing practices across cultures impact the level of independence or inter-reliance that is fostered from early childhood. The child's desire for mastery and the environment's demand for mastery are sometimes consonant and sometimes dissonant. The developing child, desiring to experience mastery and increase relative influence over interactions with the environment, must adapt to satisfy their own needs for mastery while also satisfying the contextually specific environmental expectations. The interaction of these two demands becomes the press for mastery.

The case of The Playmate (Case 2-1) illustrates the delicate balance of desire, demand, and press for a very young child with Down syndrome. Notice how the therapist carefully adjusted her expectations and used the social environment, as well as objects, to tap into the child's desires for mastery.

CASE 2-1

The Playmate

One of my most memorable early intervention clients was Ginger, a young female with Down syndrome. She was approximately 12 months old when we started working together and more than 24 months old when we stopped. I saw her at home, twice a week for 45 minutes initially and then less frequently as she progressed. She had three older brothers—ages 6, 4, and 2 (like stair steps)—who were my best friends. Her parents, both physicians, were loving and devoted parents to all their children.

Ginger was very sensitive to external demands, particularly those arising from her battery of therapists (she received occupational, physical, and speech therapies and special education services in the home weekly). Although nonverbal, she could communicate her disinterest—and displeasure—clearly. Suddenly, it was like you were no longer in the room, possibly not even in existence. All interaction ceased. Eye contact dropped, smiles evaporated, and verbalizing quieted. She turned her back and shut you out.

To prevent being shut out, I had to stay on the tips of my therapist toes, constantly learning new strategies to keep her engaged. Her brothers were enormously helpful in this effort. If I played with them and not her, she became interested and motivated again in her desire to be included. On days the boys were not there, I worked very hard indeed.

At a certain point, I was eager to get Ginger interested in stringing and unstringing jumbo wooden beads on a thick cord. I reasoned that engaging in this simple bead stringing activity would capitalize on Ginger's visual-spatial processing strength while developing her motor skills so she could better participate in preschool. She was performing well at motor tasks and had just mastered intentional drop release with less than a 12- month delay. Bead stringing would be a challenge, and I knew it would take some time. I also knew that if I brought in a set of beads and plunked it down in front of her, she would feel pressured to perform and resist play. I decided to make a necklace out of three or four of the beads in different shapes and colors and wear the necklace to therapy as part of my outfit.

I wore the necklace at least three times, never once offering it to her or bringing it to her attention before she attended to it in any way. Finally, she took the bait. Ginger wanted to play with the beads. After this, it became a routine for me to wear the necklace and for her to play with it. It took ages before she had any interest in working the beads first off and then on to the string, but she got there gradually.

This case study illustrates how the context of therapy as an occupational environment can inadvertently serve to thwart this phase of the occupational adaptation process. The good overall progress this child made in therapy is evidence she possessed a desire for mastery. Yet, the demand for mastery led her to withdraw from the interaction. Although unable to articulate it, this little girl recognized that in the context of her therapy session, her interactions with me as her therapist (although taking place in her home environment and centered around play) cast her in a different role than when she was playing at home with her family members. She also sensed this role came with very specific occupational demands. Instead of creating a press for mastery, her perception of these demands thwarted the expression of her desire for mastery, perhaps in part because this role was contrived, and she was not innately motivated to fulfill it. Her self-identity included a child who plays but did not include a child who engages in therapy.

When the demand for mastery was modified (decreased), the child's desire for mastery was activated. Her adaptive process relied on reducing the environmental demand (my expectations as her therapist that she perform well on therapeutic activities) until the press stimulated (rather than thwarted) her desire. In other words, when our interactions felt like child-directed play instead of adult-directed therapy, it was fun again, and her desire was engaged with the press for mastery in the form of a just-right challenge.

Case contributed by Kyle Karen, MS, PhD

Press for Mastery Over the Life Span

The press for mastery continues over a lifetime. Factors over which we wish to exert influence change over time. Environmental demands also change, but the need to respond adaptively and masterfully continues. Occupational challenges occur in different locations and contexts, but they do not go away. An important thing to remember is that we move in and out of occupational performance situations in which we feel competent. Even very competent people can feel unsure when confronted with significant challenges. Nevertheless, the press for mastery exists with interaction from both the person and the environment.

Now, let us consider the story of The Sixth Grade Student (Story 2-1) whose levels of adaptation were shaken under imposed environmental restrictions because of the coronavirus disease 2019 (COVID-19) pandemic. This story illustrates how a change in the environment can create a wide range of demands on a person, each requiring an adaptive response.

To further illustrate the impact of the environment's demands for mastery, let us explore the example of a teacher who has been working successfully in elementary education for 30 years and must confront new challenges in light of COVID-19 restrictions on in-person instruction. This teacher is competent in the classroom. She creates an atmosphere that is conducive to learning, where the children feel valued and accepted. She knows what students can and cannot do. She knows how to provide instruction that reaches every child on a level each can handle. She takes pride in her high-quality work (desire for mastery). Suddenly, she must ensure that her students produce excellent work while learning in an online (virtual) environment. The principal and parents want her to continue producing high-quality learning outcomes in the same subject areas (demand for mastery). The resulting press for mastery means that she must adapt to increased use of online learning platforms, lessons interrupted by spotty Wi-Fi signals, and navigating classroom management through a screen. The important assumption for occupational adaptation is that the desire for mastery, the demand for mastery, and the press for mastery are constants when striving for competence in occupational functioning even when circumstances change.

Organizational or process changes in work situations are everywhere. Reorganization, downsizing, managed care, and reimbursement changes in health care are powerful examples that therapists encounter daily. The dynamic tension between the professional desires of the therapist and the health care system can intensify. Nevertheless, therapists wish to respond adaptively and masterfully for the benefit of their clients and the security of their jobs. The employer also expects that each therapist will respond adaptively and masterfully for the benefit of clients and the organization.

It is easy for therapists to assume that clients do not have a desire for mastery. Recall the knitter in Chapter 1 who did not make significant progress until a meaningful (motivating and desirable) role was discovered. The case of The Afghan Maker (Case 2-2) also illustrates the potential therapeutic error that can result from an assumption of no desire for mastery.

The key to occupational engagement for Mrs. Turner was creating an environment that allowed her to fulfill her desire for mastery. We might even go as far as to say that she had been in a state of occupational deprivation, with a lack of support for meaningful occupation. Occupational deprivation is an issue of occupational justice that is not always as easily identified and remedied as it was in this case.

Jennifer Whittaker, an occupational therapy practitioner and PhD student, interviewed Dr. Laurie Stelter who is an occupational therapy practitioner, researcher, educator, and noted expert in occupational adaptation. Stelter described using participatory occupational justice as the overarching theory that guided her to work with the population of women with intellectual and developmental disabilities who are incarcerated (Stelter & Evetts, 2020). She explained that occupational adaptation was the theory that laid out the process of what to do and how to do it, more specifically to "promote adaptive responses and relative mastery" with individuals in this marginalized population. She further explained that the context where the women lived (in prison) limited the demand for mastery, which affected both the desire and press for mastery, causing occupational deprivation and injustice (L. Stelter, personal communication, March 29, 2019). Whittaker's reflection on this interview provides a compelling argument for integrating an occupational justice framework into occupational therapy practice:

> Therapists knowledgeable in the tenets of occupational adaptation should take on an occupational justice framework as well. Those who believe that everyone has a desire for mastery should work explicitly to ensure that everyone also has the opportunity to fulfill that desire through living in contexts that provide just-right demands for mastery. Stelter developed a program for incarcerated women with IDD [intellectual and developmental disabilities] which aimed to do just that by expanding opportunities for participation in occupation in an environment that took away such liberties. (J. Whittaker, personal communication, March 29, 2019)

STORY 2-1

The Sixth Grade Student

As society entered shelter-in-place (a period in 2020 when businesses and schools closed most in-person operations because of the COVID-19 pandemic), our daily lives changed. As a parent, I witnessed firsthand how this affected my children and their roles as students. Although they had already achieved mastery in student roles, the disruption created major transitions that increased demands for occupational adaptation. My son had to adapt to his changed occupational role as a student during his final months in sixth grade.

The occupational environment was significantly disrupted, including the learning context, location, and method of instruction. Changes included the physical location of where he went to school, the social aspect of interacting with peers and teachers, and the cultural aspect of learning within a physical classroom environment. Learning was all virtual. Furthermore, his role as a child engaging in play and leisure activities was challenged. The physical location where he engaged in play along with the social aspect with peers and the associated cultural norms were all interrupted. Play and leisure activities with peers using specific objects, engaging in social participation, and following rules they laid out (e.g., playing three-on-three basketball) were no longer accessible in the same manner.

His self-care was also disrupted. However, in his case, he reported it as something positive. He had access to food all day, could wear comfortable clothing without shoes, and did not have to ask for permission to go to the bathroom. He also enjoyed the fact that he could relax on the couch when he felt eyestrain or sit out on the balcony to get fresh air.

The changing environment impacted the configuration of his person–system gestalt. The use of his motor skills was affected because of a shift that significantly decreased demands for physical activity. The shelter-in-place no longer required him to walk around to change classes nor enabled him to run around during recess or engage in physical activities during physical education class. He no longer had the same access to experiential learning due to altered ability to physically see, hear, or touch to enhance learning.

His process skills were over-ridden by the emotional impact of isolation from his peers. The change in the environment created such a dramatic shift that it affected him on an emotional level. There was a decline in his quality of work, he was late submitting assignments, and he was also frustrated by the amount of screen time he had to tolerate daily.

In this scenario, the occupational environment created a demand for mastery (continue to make good grades in the changing learning environment), and the student's desire for mastery (wanting to advance to the next grade) was strong. The resulting occupational challenge of completing schoolwork in a virtual environment is where the press for mastery occurred. As a result of a change in his personal and environmental contexts, an occupational challenge emerged that influenced his occupational role expectations and experience of relative mastery.

Story contributed by Alondra Ammon, MOT, OTR/L

RESEARCH QUESTION

Consider the following researchable question: What is the impact on overall health and well-being when an extended period of occupational deprivation is interrupted with opportunity for meaningful occupation? This question can be applied to individuals, groups, or populations, including parolees, immigrants granted asylum, those released from prolonged hospitalization, and institutionalized residents introduced to new programming. How might you go about tapping into the desire for mastery and providing opportunities to engage in just-right challenges for people in your community? How might you design a research study to document change?

CASE 2-2 ———

The Afghan Maker

The following case is a result of two occupational therapy students serving a client in a nursing home as part of their fieldwork practice. Their clinical reasoning and theoretical considerations were reflected in a written summary after class treatment team discussions.

Mrs. Turner was an 84-year-old woman living in a nursing home. Her chart indicated she had been discharged from occupational therapy services on two previous occasions secondary to refusal to participate. Before seeing Mrs. Turner, the students assumed that she did not have a desire for mastery because of her limited participation in activities and her documented decline in cognitive status.

During the initial session, the students assessed Mrs. Turner's interests. She had few active interests; however, she did recall crocheting with strong participation in the past. The students reasoned that their client was isolating herself in her room and would benefit from leaving her room to participate in other home activities. Mrs. Turner adamantly refused to leave her room or work to improve self-care as requested by the nursing staff. The students attempted several cognitive activities designed to address her memory and orientation. Although these activities involved current events and card games, Mrs. Turner demonstrated marginal engagement and limited attention span. The students finally reasoned that Mrs. Turner's past interests were the way to go. They left a ball of light blue yarn and crochet hook with her at the end of their session with the hopes of enticing interest in their next session. The next week when they returned, Mrs. Turner had not only crocheted a circular medallion with the light blue yarn, but she had also managed to secure multiple colors of yarn and showed off a crocheted mini-afghan! Mrs. Turner demonstrated various stitch patterns to the students and showed increased initiation, as evidenced by verbalizing a plan to find yellow yarn to finish it off.

This case demonstrates that the students' assumption that Mrs. Turner did not have a desire for mastery was false. The implications for practice are that a therapist must always assume that a desire for mastery is present. The occupational therapist must explore possibilities until the client's desire for mastery is identified.

Case contributed by Stephanie Springfield, OTS and Nanette Tabani, OTS

A Deeper Dive

Here is what we believe about hope. See if this explanation can be applied to what you view as hopeful.

Occupational adaptation theory asserts that all people have a desire for mastery or hope. It is crucial that when people appear hopeless, we help them discover their innate desire for mastery (i.e., "What do you want to do?"). When the desire for mastery is matched with a just-right challenge in the form of a meaningful occupational activity or task, we facilitate a successful adaptive response to the challenge so that the person can experience a sense of relative mastery. Relative mastery and success in meeting challenges sparks a cycle of desire and hope with motivation to take on the next challenge.

It is not enough to simply say "just do something" if the goal is to re-energize occupational engagement. So, how do we address hope or hopelessness? We address intervention thoroughly in Chapter 10. To get you started thinking about intervention, we suggest you investigate what your client wants to do and set up a success-oriented just-right challenge. Provide prompts and ask questions to promote adaptive responses, but intervene with your own answers or doing *only* at the point of complete frustration so that the person can own their experience of success. Do not limit your intervention tasks to a checklist of biomechanical or activities of daily living performance demands. Follow the person's interests, making it clear how any occupational readiness activities will lead toward their desired occupations. The biomechanical and/or activities of daily living improvements will follow as more hope returns.

TAKE-AWAY MESSAGES

◊ The desire for mastery is always present, even if untapped. The therapist must persist in identifying the client's underlying desire so that an opportunity for press can be orchestrated.

◊ The environment creates a demand for mastery that will surely shift over time, place, and circumstance. The therapist needs to be acutely aware of these demands to be an agent of the environment in the adaptation process.

◊ Press for mastery comes in the form of an occupational challenge. The person has an opportunity for success when there is a just-right challenge—one that matches the person's desire and modulates the environmental demands.

◊ Occupational deprivation results when no opportunities exist to engage in a desired occupation.

References

Cohn, E. S. (2019). Asserting our competence and affirming the value of occupation with confidence (Eleanor Clarke Slagle lecture). *American Journal of Occupational Therapy, 73,* 7306150010. https://doi.org/10.5014/ajot.2019.736002

Silverstein, S. (2014). Early bird. *Where the sidewalk ends* (p. 30). Harper Collins.

Stelter, L. D., & Evetts, C. L. (2020). Effect of an occupation-based program for women with intellectual and developmental disabilities who are incarcerated. *Annals of International Occupational Therapy, 3*(4), 175-184. https://doi.org/10.3928/24761222-20190910-01

Try It On

Now that we have laid some of the foundational concepts, it is time to "try it on" yourself. To begin, identify an event in your life that produced a need for you to behave adaptively and affected your ability to function adaptively. We will ask you to think about this example throughout the book as the occupational adaptation process unfolds. Maybe your event occurred as you transitioned into a new position at work, purchased a new home, or adjusted to your favorite leisure activity following an injury or age-related changes. As you contemplate your life event, think about how your desire for mastery and the environment's demand for mastery were expressed.

Life event:

Person	Environment
Why did you desire to have mastery in this situation?	How did the environment make its demands known? (Consider whether and how physical, social, or cultural contexts influenced your event.)

CHAPTER 3

Occupational Challenge, Internal and External Expectations, Person, and Occupational Environment

Where Do Occupational Role Expectations Fit?

… You have fully fathomed the depth of this calling
when your understanding starts with each story …
—Charles Christiansen (2019)

An occupational challenge is experienced in the context of an occupational role when internal desire and external demand create a press for mastery in the form of an occupation that requires an adaptive response. Occupational challenges emerge from occupational roles and the interactions between expectations associated with these roles. It is the occupational role expectations that produce the need for the occupational adaptation process to go to work. Therefore, occupational role expectations are central to occupational adaptation. You may notice that all the cases and stories in this book are titled by the occupational role that is central to the occupational adaptation process. We have found that when no discernible occupational role is apparent in a story or case report, the report usually ends in a dysadaptive state. So, we emphasize again the importance of identifying a meaningful occupational role on which to base the therapeutic intervention.

Occupational role expectations are driven by the entire context, with two primary sources: person-generated internal expectations and environment-generated external expectations. To understand how to interpret these expectations and anticipate their impact on adaptive responses, we must look at how occupational adaptation views the person and the environment and then (as Dr. Charles Christiansen reminds us) listen carefully to each client's story.

Evetts, C. L., & Baxter, M. F. *Cases and Concepts in Occupational Adaptation: Translating Theory into Action* (pp. 17-30).
DOI: 10.4324/9781003522850-3

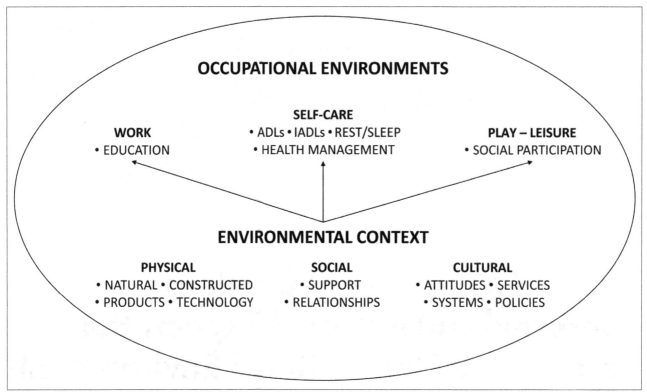

Figure 3-1. Occupational environments and influences of environmental factors in context. ADLs = activities of daily living; IADLs = instrumental activities of daily living.

The Occupational Environment and External Expectations

The occupational environment is the context in which a particular occupational role is carried out. There are many ways to think about this context. Occupational adaptation originally stated that occupational environments are work, leisure/play, or self-care. These are familiar ideas in occupational therapy and ones that come naturally to occupational therapists. Although occupational environments in general can be categorized this way, the specific features of a particular occupational environment are highly individualized. For example, your work circumstances may be very different from that of a professional friend even though you are both occupational therapists. These differences arise from various factors, including external expectations that influence each work environment in unique ways. The fourth edition of the *Occupational Therapy Practice Framework: Domain and Process* (OTPF-4) categorizes the environmental factors in our context as the natural environment (including any human-made changes); products and technology; support and relationships; attitudes; and services, systems, and policies. Together, these environmental factors represent the human and nonhuman elements within any occupational environment. The same thing can be said of the environments in

which any occupation takes place, including activities of daily living, instrumental activities of daily living, work, health management, rest and sleep, education, work, play, leisure, and social participation.

Figure 3-1 shows the occupational environments with potential influences from environmental factors in context. As we go forward, we refer to the environmental factors more broadly as physical, social, and cultural while acknowledging the complexities and nuances of context as described in the *OTPF-4*.

The environment in which a particular occupation takes place supplies the external occupational role expectations. For example, suppose one of your favorite leisure occupations is attending professional baseball games. How you carry out your role as a spectator will be influenced by the physical features of the parking lot, stadium, seats, locations of restrooms and concession stands, and so on. Friends or family who attend the game with you, the people seated around you, and those who stand in line with you are all environmental factors in this context. If you are a parent accompanying children, the social expectations will be different than on occasions when you are attending the game with adults only. Attitudes including cultural influences, customs, rules and regulations, mission, and purpose all impact occupational participation in a setting. For example, the seventh-inning stretch is an attitudinal norm, as is cheering for the home team, and playing the national anthem to begin the event is a time-honored ritual.

These environmental factors tell us what the external role expectations are in a particular situation. The specifics will differ among occupational environments, but the same principle applies. The totality of one's environment will have a tremendous impact on the occupational role choices it affords. Take under consideration the story of The Wishful Skier (Story 3-1) and the playful depiction seen in Figure 3-2.

Some have argued that assigning roles to individuals puts them at risk for ridicule or disappointment, particularly when disability or dysfunction prevents them from meeting society's expectations (Bonsall, 2019). Assigning roles and tasks is also contrary to the belief that internal desire, with accompanying internal expectations, is what leads to adaptive responses in required and desired occupational roles.

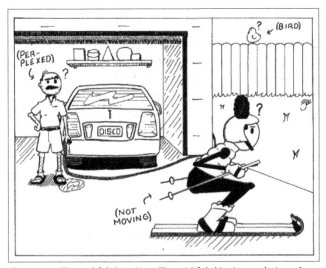

Figure 3-2. The wishful skier. *Note:* The wishful skier is wondering what the hype about skiing is all about, but the context is entirely wrong for the sport regardless of having the proper equipment and clothing. In short, context matters. (Illustrated by Mitchell Reid.)

The Person and Internal Expectations

In addition to external expectations, the individual brings their own set of internal expectations to any occupational challenge. So, how does occupational adaptation view the individual? Once again, familiar occupational therapy ideas apply. The *OTPF-4* describes the following personal factors that contribute to the context of occupational participation: age, sexual orientation, gender identity, race and ethnicity, cultural identification and cultural attitudes, social background (including social status and socioeconomic status), upbringing and life experiences, habits and behavioral patterns, psychological assets, education, profession and professional identify, lifestyle, and health conditions and fitness (American Occupational Therapy Association, 2020). Just as each opportunity for occupational participation has unique features because of the influences of environmental factors, each individual has unique personal factors contributing to their potential for occupational engagement (Figure 3-3).

In addition, genetic and familial factors classified as body functions and body structures can also have a powerful influence on the individual's internal role expectations. For example, tasks that favor having a certain physiological feature, such as a small body and a well-coordinated sensorimotor system, will not result in very positive internal role expectations if the body is large and poorly coordinated. Likewise, one's current or enduring environmental circumstances can predispose the individual to certain internal expectations. If a task requires economic or social resources that are unavailable, expectations will be influenced by that situation. Similarly, the individual's history or experience adds a phenomenological quality to the picture along with established performance patterns (roles, routines, habits, and rituals).

STORY 3-1

The Wishful Skier

There are several reasons I have never gone skiing, and foremost, is the fact that I live in the middle of Ohio. Although it snows here, the frequency is insufficient to sustain outdoor winter sporting businesses. Furthermore, the flat landscape is incongruent with the enterprise. While admittedly I lack the inner drive to take up skiing, one could also argue that my environment never presented the demand for developing skiing skills. Environmental factors are central to the adaptation process. Opportunities and challenges afforded by the environment compel individuals toward mastery or facilitate complacency. Traveling to Colorado might prompt me to try on a pair of skis; I might even benefit from the interaction, expanding my horizons by venturing into a new challenge in unfamiliar territory.

Story contributed by Brooke King, MSOT, OTR/L

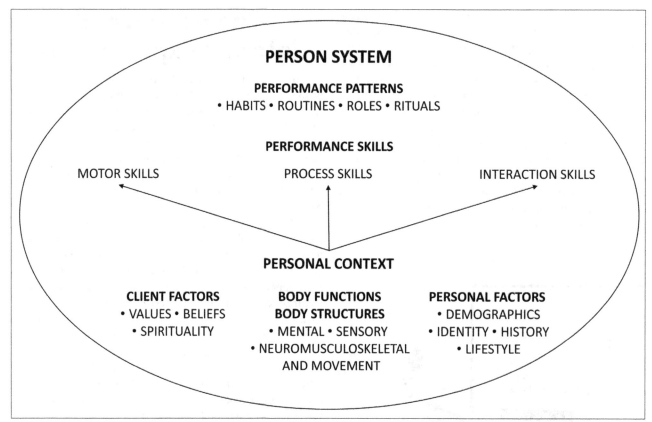

Figure 3-3. Person system. *Note:* Personal context greatly influences and enables or restricts occupational performance patterns and skills.

If the experiences have been positive, the expectations are more positive. If experiences have been negative, the expectations will likely be more negative. All these influences will impact our assessment of the likely outcomes and therefore give rise to a unique set of internal role expectations when confronting an occupational challenge.

Occupational scientist and therapist Dr. Ann Wilcock describes occupation as a synthesis of doing, being, and becoming. Occupational dysfunction is normative, not exclusively a medical issue; "…becoming through doing and being is part of daily life for all people on earth not just those in hospital or health centre" (Wilcock, 1999, p. 6). She also sees occupational roles as central to identity, health, and well-being and cautions us to be aware of potentially harmful external expectations that are unwanted or unrealistic.

> Indeed, we tend to imbue the state of being with the notions of doing particularly when we use it to describe occupational roles as in being a parent, being a student, being a sportsperson, or being an occupational therapist. While the notion of being is important to us in this way, the cultural drives to do better and better alters ways of being in particular roles and overwhelms with a huge range of beings in each of which we are expected to become perfect. (Wilcock, 1999, p. 5)

To heed Dr. Wilcock's warning, we focus on understanding each client's story and personal perspective, including their unique occupational role expectations.

The case of The Retired Yoga Instructor (Case 3-1) illustrates how long-held internal expectations and an immediate desire for mastery drive this plucky friend toward an adaptive response. Notice how she draws on her personal experience in new ways to adapt to a challenging situation.

Occupational Challenge and Interacting Expectations

Thus, the occupational challenges presented to the individual are embedded within roles, which include expectations that are idiosyncratic to the individual performing within a particular environmental context. For example, although there are common attributes within the parent role (i.e., care for the survival and developmental needs of one's children), there are substantial differences that stem from the physical, social, and cultural demands of the specific occupational environment in which the parental role encounters a challenge. A parent responding to the behavior of a child

CASE 3-1 ─────────────────────────────────────

The Retired Yoga Instructor

My client was a 70-year-old woman seen in an outpatient setting. Ms. Bergamont had broken her left hip and had it repaired by anterior total hip arthroplasty. Her occupational challenge was rising from sit to stand from a low surface without adaptive equipment. While at the skilled nursing facility, she learned to rise from higher surfaces and to use external support, such as using a raised commode seat and toilet rails. However, she reported having difficulty with the transitional movement of sit to stand from a low toilet seat at her friend's house the prior Sunday. She had previously been a yoga instructor and lamented that she used to be able to bend to touch the floor and come up to a standing position easily. With the occupational therapist's guidance, the client placed her hands on the floor from a sitting position and rose to standing with her arms above her head in a movement that approximated the one she had practiced for many years during yoga. Ms. Bergamont repeated the process several times, achieving a renewed sense of relative mastery after several repetitions and gaining confidence to continue to engage socially at her friend's house.

One concept illustrated by Ms. Bergamont is how the occupational environment presents a demand for mastery. Within the contexts and intersections of leisure and self-care, we see these factors at play. The physical environment significantly included a lower toilet seat than the client had encountered since her hip surgery and the absence of toilet rails or grab bars. Culturally, Ms. Bergamont is originally from England and values modesty to a great degree. Additionally, she is an older Caucasian woman in the southwestern United States, and the culture prizes independence and youth. Therefore, it goes against cultural norms for people to be open about physical limitations or difficulty performing self-care tasks independently. Prevailing attitudes demand that friendships function under these norms and maintain boundaries accordingly. As such, it seemed inappropriate to Ms. Bergamont to request assistance getting off the toilet seat from her friend, so she sat on the toilet for approximately 20 minutes before being able to finally rise, which was completely unsatisfactory. This situation created a demand for mastery and, when combined with the client's desire for mastery, contributed to the formation of the press for mastery, which ultimately produced an adaptive response to this unique occupational challenge.

Case contributed by Lindsay Ballew, MOT, OTR/L

who has violated a rule of the household is in a very different position from the parent who responds to a teacher's request for a conference based on that same child's failure to perform satisfactorily in the school environment. Both situations involve the parental role, but the environmental contexts within which these challenges must be confronted are distinctively different.

The next case provides you with an opportunity to examine the environmental demands on an infant and her family in the cardiovascular intensive care unit (Case 3-2). Notice how the therapist addresses the challenges of both the infant and her parents. In this situation, the infant, mom, dad, and therapists each have their challenges while each contributes to the occupational environment of the others.

For the therapist, the importance of role expectations is that they become the structure on which you plan and implement intervention with the collaboration of the client. The client may have to help you understand those expectations

when the role is unfamiliar to you or expectations are environmentally different from your own experience. Role-related occupational challenges may range from minor in scope and temporary in duration to major in scope and of extended duration. Conceptualizing expectations is important whether your focus is on an individual who is experiencing those minor/temporary challenges expected as a part of living, one with major but temporarily disruptive challenges, or one with chronic disabling conditions that result in major and persistent challenges (Figure 3-4).

Once again, the therapist must not assume that they know the occupational role expectations for a particular client. In many cases, the client becomes the teacher and the therapist the learner. This relationship sets the stage for true collaboration between the client and the therapist. The client brings their knowledge of the expectations, and the therapist brings their expertise in occupational functioning.

NEURO SPOTLIGHT

Desire, Demand, and Press

Desire, demand, and press for mastery (also known as *motivation*) are essential to survival, learning, well-being, and the generation of goal-directed occupations. Desire, demand, and press are modulated by many different and interconnected neurologic structures and functions. Additionally, there are various sources and types of motivation. Desire for mastery includes all the varied motivational forces that we encounter, including implicit and objective (e.g., thirst and hunger) demands, and motivational forces that are conscious and cognitive (e.g., intrinsic motivation and attaining ultimate goals). Desire for mastery results from environment requirements and demands and requires that behaviors or actions that maximize the chances of survival are selectively identified and engaged.

Desire for mastery that is implicit and objective appears to be linked to the autonomic nervous system, homeostasis, and emotional regulation. Emotional regulation is processed through the frontal lobe/anterior cingulate gyrus, the dorsolateral frontal lobe, the amygdala/anterior temporal regions, and the cerebellum. Literature indicates that there are some slight differences in right vs. left lobe processing for positive and negative emotions, respectively.

Higher levels of desire for mastery, such as conscious decision making, goal attainment, and intrinsic motivation, involve complex interactions with cognitive, affective, and behavioral processes and are mediated by multiple neural structures and connections. In fact, there are at least 15 key brain structures that are spread throughout the cerebral cortex that mediate desire for mastery. Five structures reside within the neocortex: the prefrontal cortex, ventromedial prefrontal cortex, dorsolateral prefrontal cortex, orbitofrontal cortex, and anterior cingulate cortex. There are six structures of the basal ganglia, including the striatum, caudate nucleus, putamen, ventral striatum nucleus, accumbens, and globus pallidus, and there are four structures that are part of the limbic system (i.e., amygdala, hypothalamus, hippocampus, insular cortex).

Additionally, understanding the neurobiology of desire for mastery requires looking at the neurotransmitter systems that support and process desire for mastery. Dopamine is the primary neurotransmitter of desire for mastery. Indeed, dopamine is associated with cognitive flexibility, increased positive affect, and creativity, which contribute to desire for mastery.

Demand for mastery results from environmental challenges and demands that are encountered in daily living and requires that behaviors or actions that maximize the chances of survival are selectively identified and engaged. This demand for mastery requires selectively or collectively using all five senses and also other bodily senses, including proprioception and vestibular functioning for continual monitoring of any perceived opportunities or hazards in the environment. Neurologic structures and processes that support demand for mastery begin with the structures that receive environmental input, such as the eyes, ears, vestibular apparatus, and receptors in joints and muscles that contribute to proprioception. The neurologic processes will then depend on the sensations that are being used either singly or in combination. Demand for mastery, like desire for mastery, is mediated by dopaminergic neurotransmitters.

Press for mastery brings together the desires and the demands for mastery and involves complex neurologic processes across multiple neural structures. Because internal and external conditions fluctuate dynamically and often unpredictably, the adaptation and selection of behaviors must be performed quickly and flexibly to adapt to the individual desires or needs and the demands of the environment. Therefore, a multitude of central nervous system structures and processes are involved in the press for mastery.

(continued)

Additionally, the neurologic substrates for desire, demand, and press for mastery appear to be associated with whether the demand or the task requires more physical effort or cognitive effort. Desire, demand, and press for mastery that require physical effort are primarily processed through the limbic system and the ventral striatum and pallidum of the basal ganglia with primary connections to the motor cortex. Cognitive effort is processed through connections from the ventral prefrontal cortex to the ventral striatum in the basal ganglia. The ventral striatum then contributes to or modulates the motor or cognitive divisions of the dorsal striatum depending on the task. There is also a connection between the ventral striatum and the dorsal striatum that is common for the demand, desire, or press for mastery of cognitive and physical effort in a task or goal-directed behavior.

In summary, demand, desire, and press for mastery are intertwined processes that involve complicated connections with each other and with many neurologic structures and functions. Consequently, impairment in any cerebral structure can affect demand, desire, or press for mastery in myriad ways.

RECOMMENDED READINGS

Di Domenico, S. I., & Ryan, R. M. (2017). The emerging neuroscience of intrinsic motivation: A new frontier in self-determination research. *Frontiers in Human Neuroscience, 11*, 145. https://doi.org/10.3389/fnhum.2017.00145

Simpson, E. H., & Balsam, P. D. (2016). The behavioral neuroscience of motivation: An overview of concepts, measures, and translational applications. *Current Topics in Behavioral Neurosciences, 27*, 1-12. https://doi.org/10.1007/7854_2015_402

CASE 3-2

The New Family

Upon entering the room of a 2-day-old infant with a diagnosis of hypoplastic left heart syndrome, the following observations were made:

- Noise: Medical staff rounding bedside and speaking loudly with alarms going off secondary to a lead placed incorrectly and autonomic instability.
- Lighting: Bright, direct light was placed overhead by staff during evaluation.
- State of infant: The infant was unswaddled with staff looking at the peripherally inserted central catheter dressing and evaluating heart sounds. She was exhibiting signs of distress including extension of both upper and lower extremities, color changes, and autonomic changes of increased heart rate and decreased oxygen saturation.
- State of caregiver: Mom was sitting in a wheelchair across the room in obvious distress. This was her first time visiting her infant after delivery; she had been brought by medical staff from the hospital where she had given birth.

The environment was contributing to a dysadaptive response by the new family, both the infant and the parents. Once the medical staff concluded their evaluation, discussed the medical plan with the mom and dad, and left the room, the therapist assisted the infant and caregiver in the following ways to create less of an environmental demand and an increased adaptive response to their situation:

- Noise: Alarms were silenced, and leads were correctly placed. The remaining staff were asked to quiet their voices.
- Lighting: Direct overhead lighting was extinguished. Blinds were opened to let in diffuse natural light.
- Infant: Deep pressure was applied to the infant's head and body; once calmed, she was swaddled with her hands to midline near her face to provide containment.

(continued)

24   Chapter 3

- Caregiver: The parents were provided with education regarding how the environment can impact their infant's responses in both positive and negative ways. They were shown what they could do to calm and provide comfort for their infant and were given a list of things that they could currently do to bond and provide special care to their baby. Mom was immediately interested in kangaroo care and holding; the occupational therapist assisted with all lines and tubes for the mom to hold her infant. Before holding, the mom was able to change her infant's diaper and was shown how to keep her upper extremities swaddled and contained during the change to provide her with extra support during a potentially stressful time for the infant. A privacy screen was provided for the family so they could have time bonding without interruption.

At the end of the intervention, both the infant and the caregivers were calm and happy. The infant's heart rate and oxygen saturation had returned to within normal limits, she was in a light sleep state, and she had brought her hand to her mouth. Mom was smiling and singing to the baby, and dad was sitting next to mom, talking to the infant.

The parents' desire for mastery is to protect and nurture their child and create a happy family. The infant's desire for mastery can be described as the desire to attract positive attention, eat, and sleep in an environment that is safe and nurturing. The environment in the cardiovascular intensive care unit is daunting to parents and often presents demands on the infant that are incongruous with the infant's abilities. Bright lights, loud noises, inconsistent schedules, and frequent painful medical care are demands presented by the environment that the infant is not developmentally prepared to handle. As such, it has been my observation that staff must be aware and create an environment where the demand is not more than the infant can assume.

Case contributed by Stefanie Casey Rogers, PhD, OTR

OCCUPATIONAL CHALLENGE	Minor	Major
Temporary Duration	Going for a training run; favorite running socks are in the dirty laundry hamper	Traveled to run in a race; forgot to pack running socks
Extended Duration	Developed an allergy to favorite brand of wool running socks	Foot amputated due to peripheral artery disease; must wear clean stump socks with prosthesis

Figure 3-4. Occupational challenge: no clean socks. *Note:* A competitive runner with diabetes has repeated occupational challenges due to the necessity of having clean socks.

Attention to the occupational role demands as the client experiences them can lead to an effective and satisfying outcome for all concerned. It also empowers the client to be an active, collaborative participant in the therapeutic process.

We hope that the importance of understanding the complete context surrounding an occupational challenge is clear. Next, we present the case of The Video Gamer (Case 3-3) followed by some questions to help you apply what you have learned so far. You may want to have a copy of the Case 3-3 Worksheet and the *OTPF-4* handy as a guide to make sure you consider all aspects of the context as described. As you read, make a list of any words, diagnoses, abbreviations, or processes that you need to look up to fully grasp this scenario.

CASE 3-3

The Video Gamer

MEDICAL HISTORY

Charlie is a 9-year-old boy who was postnatally diagnosed with tetralogy of Fallot with pulmonary atresia, right aortic arch, and bilateral superior vena cava draining to the coronary sinus. Charlie is now status post–right ventricle to pulmonary artery conduit change, atrial septal defect closure, and pulmonary angioplasty. This is Charlie's third heart surgery since birth, and he has had multiple hospital admissions for heart catheterizations and other heart-related issues.

SOCIAL HISTORY

Charlie is an only child who is homeschooled by his mom. Charlie's mom reported that he had therapies in the past from age 8 months to 16 months, but she was unsure whether they were occupational, physical, or speech therapies. She did state that the primary goals were feeding and swallowing. Charlie had a gastrostomy tube for nutrition in the past but was currently an oral feeder. Mom also revealed that Charlie had difficulty with handwriting, was unable to ride a bicycle, was often very cautious and fearful in new environments, and had difficulty navigating uneven surfaces. Charlie exhibited a disconjugate gaze upon the occupational therapist's evaluation, and his mom said they had recommendations to alternate patching of his eyes but had been inconsistent and finally ceased. She stated they "probably need to go back and see the doctor again soon."

GENERAL APPEARANCE

Charlie was quiet and did not talk initially during the occupational therapist's evaluation. He was cooperative but did not make a lot of eye contact and refused to participate in any activities of daily living. He was in a hospital gown and in bed when the occupational therapist arrived. He also had a pulse oximeter on a finger on his right hand, telemetry leads on his chest, one chest tube, and a sternal incision.

OCCUPATIONAL ROLE ASSESSMENT

Charlie was first prompted by the occupational therapist that he was "in a children's hospital and that we have many activities and all kinds of things to do." He was then asked, "What is it that you like to do more than anything else?" Charlie identified playing video games, specifically Minecraft (Mojang Studios) and Fortnite (Epic Games). Charlie's desire for mastery was to effectively participate in his identified and preferred occupational role of a typical child-based role—playing video games.

DISCHARGE OBJECTIVES

Charlie's challenge in the inpatient acute care setting was to get out of bed, improve tolerance to activity, use his upper extremities against gravity within the limits of his sternal precautions, and perform age-appropriate activities to be able to discharge from the hospital and go home. He needed to be out of bed and moving to decrease the chest tube output for it to be removed and to achieve all the previously described activities in an unfamiliar and possibly frightening place. Charlie was afraid to move, did not want to get out of bed, and did not want to participate in any activities.

A TURNING POINT

Charlie was excited to participate in video gaming, a self-identified internally motivated activity. His demeanor instantly changed, and he began to talk about his favorite games and how good he was at them. When Charlie related with a self-identified occupational role that was familiar to him, the previously identified environmental demands were manageable and not insurmountable. Charlie began to see his environment as his room where he could participate in enjoyable activities and not an unfamiliar place with medical equipment.

(continued)

RESPONSE

Charlie was given the option of a video game system to play, which would be immediately provided by Child Life. Charlie was interested and somewhat excited by the option. Child Life was contacted to deliver the gaming system, and the game was set up across the room in front of a bedside chair. Charlie was told that he could play the game when he walked to the chair. Charlie was instantly attempting to sit up in bed and move to the edge of the bed; the occupational therapist assisted with the transition and lines/tubes. Charlie stated he was cold once he was sitting on the edge of the bed and asked to put his pajama pants on; the occupational therapist observed and gave tips for him to get dressed in compliance with his lines/tubes. Charlie performed most of the activity by himself. When the occupational therapist handed him gripper socks, he put them on independently without prompting. Charlie ambulated with standby assistance to the bedside chair and requested to use the bathroom. On the way there, the occupational therapist assisted with managing lines and tubes, but Charlie did most of the toileting activity by himself with only standby assistance. Charlie was prompted to pick a game, set up the game, and show the occupational therapist how to play. He stood for approximately 10 minutes during the setup before asking to sit down. Through self-identified role identification and participation in self-selected meaningful activity, Charlie became the agent of change and was able to participate in all the activities that would decrease his hospital length of stay.

Case contributed by Stefanie Casey Rogers, PhD, OTR

The Video Gamer Challenge

Use Case 3-3: The Video Gamer to fill out the corresponding worksheet at the end of this chapter. We hope you enjoy this challenge. When you finish, you can see our responses in the Case 3-3 Worksheet answer key in Appendix B. Do we agree? You may have insights that we overlooked or left out.

A Deeper Dive: The Vacationer

For another challenge, read the case of Sadie (Carandang & Pyatak, 2018), a college student who describes "taking a vacation" from her diabetes. Ask yourself the same basic questions that guided your review of Charlie's situation as the video gamer. What is Sadie's complete context, and how does that set expectations for her performance in her occupational roles? How are the concepts of body state and biographical moment congruent or discordant with explanations of the occupational adaptation process?

Remember that it is also crucial to understand the internal and external expectations that fuel desire and demand for mastery of a meaningful role. Notice that we did not specifically mention barriers that might impede progress. Because occupational adaptation is a strengths-based approach, we tend to focus on challenges to be responded to, rather than barriers. We think helping others see challenges as opportunities to find creative ways of responding is a more positive and encouraging stance, rather than being disappointed by encountering barriers and feeling like the environment is conspiring against us.

Next time you encounter a perceived barrier in the way of a press for mastery, ask yourself what the internal and external expectations are in the situation. The questions to consider are:

- Is there a clash between desire and demand?
- How might the expectations shift to reduce the conflict and enlighten a new way forward?

In summary, we hope that you understand the importance of working with your client to identify a meaningful occupational role to direct the intervention goals and actions.

This worksheet answer key is available in Appendix B.

TAKE-AWAY MESSAGES

◊ The full context surrounding an occupational challenge has the potential to impact both internal and external expectations for adaptive responses during occupational performance.

◊ When contextual expectations are made known, clients (persons, groups, and populations) choose whether to internalize expectations and whether to act on those internal expectations.

◊ When internal and external expectations are discordant, the occupational challenge is made more difficult.

◊ The likelihood of a successful experience with an occupational challenge is enhanced when internal and external expectations are met.

References

American Occupational Therapy Association. (2020). *Occupational therapy practice framework: Domain and process* (4th ed.). Author.

Bonsall, A. (2019). It's not a role: A conceptualization of parenting occupations [Abstract]. *Seventh Annual Proceedings of The Society for the Study of Occupation: USA* (pp. 59-60). https://www.sso-usa.net/assets/docs/proceedings_2019.pdf

Carandang, K., & Pyatak, E. A. (2018). Analyzing occupational challenges through the lens of body and biography. *Journal of Occupational Science, 25*(2), 161-173. https://doi.org/10.1080/14427591.2018.1446353

Christiansen, C. (2019). Meditation on a calling. In B. A. B. Schell, & G. Gillen (Eds.), *Willard & Spackman's occupational therapy* (13th ed., p. 1). Wolters Kluwer.

Wilcock, A. A. (1999). Reflections on doing, being, and becoming. *Australian Occupational Therapy Journal, 46*, 1-11. https://doi.org/10.1177/000841749806500501

Try It On

Recall the life event that you identified in the last chapter as providing a need for adaptation. What were the role expectations you had for yourself that made this situation an occupational challenge? What were the role expectations from the environment that contributed to the occupational challenge? Remember that the occupational challenge is a function that you need or want to carry out. Role expectations are intimately related to your desire for mastery and the environment's demand for mastery.

Occupational Challenge: _____

You: Internal Role Expectations
What did you expect of yourself in this role and the challenge it presented?

Environment: External Role Expectations
What did the environment expect of you in this role and the challenge it presented?

In the next chapter, we will ask you to continue reflecting on these expectations as we explore the internal process of how persons respond to challenges and try to meet those expectations.

CASE 3-3 WORKSHEET
The Video Gamer Challenge

List the definitions and descriptions of the words, diagnoses, abbreviations, or processes that you investigated.

Bonus: Which therapies did Charlie most likely receive before this hospitalization?

Describe Charlie's typical and immediate contexts; include both personal and environmental factors.
- Be sure to distinguish between the facts you know and the assumptions you may have made based on what you know.

TYPICAL Context: Facts (F)/Assumptions (A)	IMMEDIATE Context: Facts (F)/Assumptions (A)

- How can you confirm your suspicions? In other words, what is necessary to turn assumptions into the knowledge of facts?

Speculate on possible reasons why Charlie may have refused activities of daily living during his first meeting with the occupational therapist. Consider both internal and external expectations related to Charlie's occupational role(s).

In this scenario, what was the environmental demand for Charlie?

What was Charlie's desire?

What provided press for mastery via a just-right occupational challenge?

Bonus: Which of Charlie's favorite games would you recommend he engage in and why?

A Deeper Dive Worksheet
The Vacationer

Read Carandang, K., & Pyatak, E. A. (2018). Analyzing occupational challenges through the lens of body and biography. *Journal of Occupational Science, 25*(2), 161-173. https://doi.org/10.1080/14427591.2018.1446353.

Create a list of definitions/descriptions of the words, diagnoses, abbreviations, or processes that you need to understand better.

Describe Sadie's typical and immediate contexts; include both personal and environmental factors.
- Be sure to distinguish between what you know and the assumptions you may have made based on what you know.

TYPICAL (HOME) Context: Facts (F)/Assumptions (A)	IMMEDIATE (COLLEGE) Context: Facts (F)/Assumptions (A)

Speculate on possible reasons why Sadie may have neglected her health-maintenance role. Consider both internal and external expectations related to Sadie's occupational role(s).

In this scenario, what was the environment demanding of Sadie?

How are the concepts of body state and biographical moment congruent or discordant with explanations of the occupational adaptation process (specifically internal and external role expectations)?

Bonus: What would you recommend for Sadie and why?

Evetts, C. L., & Baxter, M. F. (2024). *Cases and Concepts in Occupational Adaptation: Translating Theory into Action.* SLACK Incorporated.

CHAPTER 4

Adaptive Response Generation, Adaptive Response Mechanism

How Does the Person Begin to Produce the Response?

---

*He started to sing as he tackled the thing
that couldn't be done, and he did it!*
—Edgar A. Guest (n.d.)

The person has a perception of the role expectations within a particular occupational challenge. The next steps are to create a response, evaluate it, and integrate it. These steps occur through the action of subprocesses within the individual's occupational adaptation process. These subprocesses are known respectively as adaptive response *generation*, adaptive response *evaluation*, and adaptive response *integration*. The functions of these subprocesses are to facilitate an adaptive response, hence their name. They do not always produce an adaptive response, just as a dysfunctional cardiovascular system may not pump blood to the extremities in a satisfactory manner. Nevertheless, the function for which the cardiovascular system exists does not change, and we do not change the name nor do we rename an adaptive response subprocess

that is dysfunctional. Each of these subprocesses exists to facilitate adaptive responses to challenges. When there is dysfunction in one or more of these subprocesses, the occupational adaptation process is dysfunctional.

The first part of this process is when the response is created or generated, thus the adaptive response generation. The next two chapters are devoted to adaptive response generation. This is an abstract idea but a very important one. It is also the most unique feature of occupational adaptation and probably its greatest contribution to occupational therapy intervention. Therefore, it is important to roll up your sleeves and wrestle with these ideas to master them. In short, this is where the real fun begins.

Evetts, C. L., & Baxter, M. F. *Cases and Concepts in Occupational Adaptation:
Translating Theory into Action* (pp. 31-46).
DOI: 10.4324/9781003522850-4

Adaptive Response Generation

For a person to generate adaptive responses, they need to have opportunities to engage in meaningful occupational challenges. If we intervene with assistance too soon or remove all obstacles to ease task completion, we take away the opportunity for our clients to learn by experience and feel masterful. It takes patience, empathy, and expressions of confidence to allow others to struggle toward personal victory—no matter how great or small.

Teri K. Rupp is an occupational adaptation scholar and an occupational therapist in school-based practice with high school students who have significant challenges with learning. She was intrigued by the idea that we need to give clients exposure to possibilities and opportunities to generate adaptive responses. She reflected on what that means for her students.

> I think [lack of opportunity to generate a response] happens a lot with my severe-profound kids, a lot of them are nonverbal, but they are obviously communicating … And I think [teachers not understanding what the student wants] ends up being a challenge for a lot of people, because they make decisions *for* them, and they do *to* them. My kids are not actors, *they are acted upon* all day long. They are never actors in their life. And so … we never let them fail. [However], they can't problem solve their way out of a paper bag because we've asked them to be compliant. And so anytime I present [a challenge]—Holy moly, I can't even get them to generate something! Their [adaptive response] generation is "I would ask somebody for help." And why is that? Because that's what we've told them to do. Since they were in second grade, when we threw them into self-contained classes, "you have a problem, you ask for help," period. (T. K. Rupp, personal communication, April 24, 2019)

Adaptive response generation is the anticipatory portion of the occupational adaptation process. From a therapeutic perspective, this anticipatory activity is where the occupational therapy intervention will need to have its ultimate impact. In other words, as a therapist, you desire that the client will be able to anticipate the outcomes of self-generated responses. Anticipating potential outcomes, both good and bad, promotes more adaptive and masterful responses. However, even infants come upon adaptive responses that are initially generated reflexively or randomly; the same can be true for children and adults. However, if we overprotect our clients, like the students at Rupp's school, and deny them an opportunity to try something on their own, they will neither adapt nor achieve mastery over occupational challenges.

Adaptive response generation consists of two components: the adaptive response mechanism and the adaptation gestalt. The adaptive response mechanism does some preliminary work in generating the response, and the adaptation gestalt plans the holistic inclusion of all that is within the person system. This chapter focuses on the adaptive response mechanism. Chapter 5 deals with the adaptation gestalt component.

Adaptive Response Mechanism

The response creation flow begins when the individual activates the adaptive response mechanism. There are three components within the adaptive response mechanism: (a) the adaptation energy that drives the process; (b) the adaptive response modes, which encompass the patterns of responding to challenges that have developed with time and experience; and (c) the adaptive response behaviors (i.e., the particular actions that the person uses in an attempt to respond adaptively). Figure 4-1 lays out the components and principal characteristics of the adaptive response mechanism. All three components of the adaptive response mechanism are active simultaneously. There is no particular order in which these components act nor is one more significant or important than the other. Do not think of them as a hierarchy. We are simply "freeze-framing" the process to understand how the adaptive response mechanism operates.

Adaptation Energy

There are two levels of adaptive energy that a person is capable of processing simultaneously or separately when engaged in occupations. Originally, Hans Selye's (1956) work on adaptation energy and general adaptation syndrome influenced the perspective of occupational adaptation. Selye's scientific work was on the impact of stress on the adrenal glands, as seen in laboratory animals. According to Selye, adaptation energy is a hypothetical quantity of energy available to use during adaptation. Selye measured the duration and intensity of adaptation energy through his work in stress adaptation and general adaptation syndrome. Although Selye has influenced the thinking about adaptation energy in occupational adaptation, the concept is understood and used differently in occupational adaptation. Additionally, research in neuroscience related to cognitive processing stress, adaptation, and resilience contributes to updated concepts of adaptation energy. Occupational adaptation proposes that the way to maximize benefits of adaptation energy is to use its two levels—primary and secondary energy—in such a way as to produce the most efficient, effective, and satisfying outcomes.

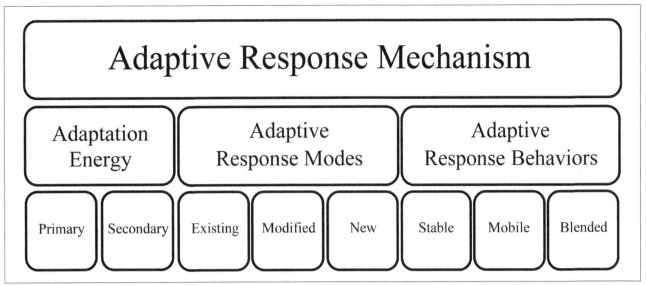

Figure 4-1. The adaptive response mechanism. *Note:* This figure does not imply a linear progression or any particular alignment of the elements. Adaptation energy, modes, and behaviors can be seen in a vast array of combinations depending on the context.

Primary adaptation energy is active when intention, volition, and focused attention are directed to the occupational challenge at hand. Imagine that you are folding an origami crane for the first time. You carefully follow the instructions, focusing intently on the task at hand; this uses primary adaptation energy. Intention, focused attention, and other higher-level cognitive functions, such as executive decision making, planning, emotional control, and problem solving, are processed generally in the frontal lobe. So, it could be suggested that primary energy as described is processed through connections in the prefrontal cortex of the frontal lobe.

Secondary adaptation energy is active when intentional and focused attention is directed away from the occupational challenge at hand and could be involved in reflection, daydreaming, self-awareness, personal emotions, long-term memory, and creativity. To build on the origami example, imagine now that you have folded so many origami cranes that you can fold the bird without any thought. As you get lost in the task, mindlessly folding while your mind wanders, you are tapping into secondary adaptation energy. Research in neuroscience related to creativity and creative thought processes indicates that inspiration, creative problem solving, reflections, and daydreaming are processed in the networks throughout the brain but appear to function more fluidly when the prefrontal cortex (primary energy) is suppressed. Nobel Prize–winning neuroscientist Santiago Ramón y Cajal (1999) offers advice to young scientists by telling them that if the solution to a problem eludes them, they should rest awhile or take a walk outside, and then possible solutions will become apparent. Think about the many times you have had a great idea or solved a particularly troublesome problem when in the shower, walking the dog, or just drifting off to sleep.

The prefrontal cortex is susceptible to stress, environmental challenges, and mental health impairments. Therefore, primary adaptation energy as processed through the prefrontal cortex can be used at a high rate. Think about when you were focused on a difficult project, were studying for a test, or were lost in a strange location. When the issue is resolved, the test is over, and when you are safe, you often experience fatigue; primary adaptation energy has been depleted temporarily. Secondary adaptation energy is processed through neural networks that are more stable and less susceptible to degradation. Therefore, secondary adaptation energy acts at a lower awareness level and uses energy at a slower rate. Think of the feelings of contentment, satisfaction, or enjoyment when you complete a creative project, mark a task off your to-do list, or engage with family on a fun project.

How do energy use and adaptive response generation relate? When we approach problem solving at the primary level, we tend to set up problem-solving structures. This can be a good strategy. However, these structures can actually limit creative problem solving when we let them restrict us to the boundaries of a particular construct. We often must work harder (using more primary energy) when we try to force solutions within boundaries. More creative and sophisticated secondary adaptation energy goes beyond the problem solution boundaries we set up when primary energy is active. The use of secondary adaptation energy leads to those sudden, creative, and insightful solutions. Because it is assumed to use less adaptation energy, secondary adaptation energy is therefore more efficient. It is logical, then, that the use of increased secondary energy is an effective tool in managing a bounded supply of energy.

When you alternate between primary energy and secondary energy, you are most likely to experience the most efficient, effective, and satisfying use of the limited supply of adaptation energy. The occupational challenge must initially be worked on at a primary level. The desired result is that the problem is then shifted or "shunted" to secondary energy. This shift of focus takes place either after primary energy activity fails to reach a solution or the demands of life send you elsewhere (e.g., to the grocery store or to walk the dog). The problem is then shunted to secondary energy for further activity while primary energy becomes directed to another task. This is somewhat like the multitasking computer environments that allow multiple projects to be worked on in parallel for greater efficiency (i.e., one program is running in the foreground while another is running in the background). For the multitasking environment to work, each of the programs must be loaded, an activity similar to working first at a primary energy level.

As an example, an occupational therapist who was one of our students was working on an important term project. This project was worth a significant percentage of the course grade. She had thought about the project a great deal. Every approach she considered (while in primary energy) seemed to lead to a dead end. Although she was skeptical about the effectiveness of the occupational adaptation principle of shunting her project to secondary energy, she decided to leave the project and knit a sweater for the infant she was expecting in a few weeks. When she completed the sweater, she returned to her project, and the elements of the project and the approach she needed to use were suddenly clear to her. In other words, secondary energy was working on her course project while primary energy worked on knitting a sweater, creating a more efficient way to reach her goal of developing the course project. With her newfound clarity on the project, all she had to do was execute the solution in written form.

This student would normally have completed her project at a primary energy level. She would have doggedly stayed on task until it was completed and expended a great deal of primary energy in the process. She would have spent more total time developing her product and bringing it to a completed written form than she did with knitting a sweater while she conceptualized her project.

This idea is not exclusive to occupational adaptation or occupational therapy. You may have heard someone comment that they were going to "put that on the back burner," meaning they were going to set an issue aside and come back to it later. Dr. Richard Carlson (1997), psychotherapist, motivational speaker, and author, encourages everyone to "experiment with your back burner" (p. 63). He especially recommends that when we are feeling stressed, it is a good time to set a problem situation aside and do something else and then come back to it later with a fresh perspective.

The metaphor of cooking and using the back burner to let something simmer is a good way to think about how secondary energy works. For example, let us consider making a pot of soup. Because good soup requires many ingredients, it takes more than boiling water to make soup; simmering alone is not enough. The proper ingredients must be assembled, prepared, and added to the pot. However, just because all the ingredients are put together, this does not guarantee a good soup. At first, the cold ingredients are adjacent to one another, but the assembly lacks cohesion that brings about blended flavors and a desired temperature; this is where the simmering comes in.

> In much the same way, we can solve many of life's problems (serious and otherwise) if we feed the back burner of our mind with a list of problems, facts, and variables, and possible solutions. Just as when we make soup or a sauce, the thoughts and ideas we feed the back of our mind must be left alone to simmer properly. (Carlson, 1997, p. 64)

Carlson (1997) asserts that shifting problems to the back of our mind "puts our quieter, softer, and sometimes most intelligent source of thinking to work for us on issues that we have no immediate answer for" (p. 64). Be cautioned that this is not an endorsement for procrastination.

You have heard some people claim that they do their best work under pressure, and therefore, they believe procrastination actually works for them. Here is the truth behind that claim; if you do the initial preparation before you set the problem or project aside, then secondary energy can work for you. However, a project set aside without any initial thoughts or preliminary plans is like simmering a pot of water with no ingredients. Even if you throw in all the right ingredients at the last minute, it will not be a well-prepared soup or project.

The construct of adaptation energy allows for an explanation of why occupation-focused intervention works to promote positive outcomes for clients we serve. Engagement in activity at a primary energy level that directs attention away from person–system deficits allows activity at the secondary energy level to produce solutions. Thus, intervention that allows the responses to emerge more automatically (less studied and focused effort) is more likely to produce the desired therapeutic outcome. The case of The Preacher (Case 4-1), based on Dolecheck and Schkade (1999) and Schultz and Schkade (1997), illustrates how a change in the therapist's approach resulted in the client's ability to use secondary energy to enhance functioning of a dysfunctional sensorimotor system while primary energy was focused on a personally meaningful occupational activity.

CASE 4-1

The Preacher

Mr. Jones was a 68-year-old African American retired minister who had suffered a stroke. He presented with characteristic neurologic damage that left him with problems in movement and speech. His multidisciplinary rehabilitation team had been concentrating intervention on the sensorimotor system (i.e., emphasis on standing tolerance, shifting his weight while standing, being able to reach across his body in diagonal patterns, speech articulation disorders). After considerable time and effort, the team had concluded that the patient was not a good candidate for walking. His documented standing tolerance was a maximum of 5 minutes, and his difficulty in weight shifting was extreme.

At this point, the therapist was introduced to occupational adaptation and the importance of focusing intervention on personally meaningful activity. In a conversation with Mr. Jones, the therapist discovered that he was a preacher and most desired to return to that occupational role. She told him that the next day she would bring a podium into the room where the Bible study group, of which Mr. Jones was a member, would meet and she wanted him to preach. Mr. Jones expressed fear and apprehension that he would not be able to preach.

The next day, a Friday, the therapist brought a podium into the room and put it in place. As soon as Mr. Jones saw this physical symbol from the occupational environment of preaching, he began to articulate a list of things he could talk about. Despite his apprehensions about standing and talking, Mr. Jones was assisted into standing and began to preach. For 20 minutes, Mr. Jones stood and preached. As he preached, he weight shifted. He gestured, crossing midline, to the full extent of his range of motion. He spoke in the most powerful voice he could summon. At the end of the 20 minutes when Mr. Jones sat down, he burst into a song, and then he cried. The following Monday, Mr. Jones began to walk.

By engaging Mr. Jones in the activity of preaching, the sensorimotor and speech deficits were shunted to secondary adaptation energy while primary energy was focused on the activity of preaching. Because the sensorimotor and speech requirements were shunted to the secondary energy for assistance, the capabilities of the sensorimotor system had been "unbound" from the structure imposed by standard protocol clinical intervention at the primary energy level. Engagement in an occupational activity that was meaningful to Mr. Jones based on the role expectations associated with preaching set the stage for him to maximize his remaining capabilities and act as his own agent of therapeutic change. Thus, the sensorimotor and speech performance requirements were able to emerge in a more automatic fashion.

Case contributed by Jessica Dolecheck, PhD, OTR (Retired)

Adaptive Response Modes

Adaptive response modes are another feature of the adaptive response mechanism. Patterns of responding to occupational challenges that have resulted in at least some degree of mastery become incorporated into the individual's adaptation repertoire (see Chapter 7) as adaptive response modes. Adaptive response modes are classified as existing (those already in our adaptive repertoire), modified (those in which we make changes in an existing mode), and new (those that come about because our existing or modified modes are not working for a particular need).

Adaptive response modes develop as an infant behaves reflexively and randomly. These reflexive and random movements sometimes produce unintentional effects on persons and objects. For example, an infant is lying in supine kicking their legs as part of the natural development of sensorimotor capability. Quite by accident, they kick a bell that is suspended above their crib. As they repeat the kicking movement and continue to experience the bell sound, they begin to make associations between these actions and certain outcomes. This is the way the adaptive response modes that produce particular outcomes become a part of the collection of familiar response patterns (Gilfoyle et al., 1990).

When confronted with an occupational challenge, our first attempt is ordinarily to use existing modes. An existing mode is one that has worked in the past; you might think "Why reinvent the wheel?" When an existing mode produces some degree of mastery, it is more efficient to use that mode because you must expend effort and adaptation energy to develop a new one. However, if the use of an existing mode does not produce some degree of mastery, there is reason to explore an alternate method. In the example of the infant kicking the bell, they may use the kicking movement in an attempt to produce some other outcome. Kicking may not have the desired effect and thus lead the infant to explore other response modes (perhaps a different movement of the leg). Sometimes a slight modification of an existing mode will produce the desired result. It is a reasonable approach to simply "tweak" an already comfortable approach, thus creating a modified mode.

I (CLE) am reminded of how my son, at age 7, wanted to understand how to balance while riding a bicycle (using primary energy). I finally convinced him to focus solely on pedaling, suggesting he "look straight ahead and forget about balancing." He learned to ride a bike, but he used his adaptation repertoire (existing adaptive response modes) to balance (learned while walking) and to steer and pedal (learned on a tricycle). Looking straight ahead at the road took up his primary energy, allowing secondary energy to generate modified behaviors (sensory and motor) and resulting in his ability to balance on a moving bicycle.

Sometimes, even substantial modification of an existing mode will not produce a satisfactory outcome. On these occasions, there is the impetus to create an entirely new pattern of interaction for an adaptive response to be realized (a new mode). The case of The Researcher (Case 4-2) illustrates how an occupational challenge can require the development of a new adaptive response mode and how the therapist facilitates the development of the new mode.

Remember that adaptive response modes are patterns of responding to environmental cues that the individual develops. Frequently, the therapist must assist a client to develop either modified or new adaptive response modes, especially when current capabilities may not allow the use of existing adaptive response modes. At the same time, the therapist might need to respond adaptively when well-established protocols are not sufficient to meet client needs. In her 2016 Eleanor Clarke Slagle lecture, Dr. Susan Garber (2016) discussed how research in the field of occupational therapy has come about when therapists become passionate about finding a better way to help a client population. When therapists are responsible for the health and safety of clients, we cannot try every idea that emerges. We must be systematic in careful experimentation to discover, document, and disseminate new knowledge about intervention that is efficient, effective, and satisfying to all who are impacted. Dr. Garber reminds us that it takes a "prepared mind" to meet the daily challenges of addressing individual and collective needs of others as an occupational therapist. Our observations tell us that the best therapists are those who continuously "feed the back burner" by staying connected to the profession through professional associations and continuing education.

Adaptive Response Behaviors

Adaptive response behaviors are the third feature of the adaptive response mechanism. Adaptive response behaviors are types of behaviors that we use in attempting to respond adaptively and masterfully. We refer to these generally as representing stable, mobile, and blended adaptive behaviors, each representing a cluster of behaviors within a continuum of potential responses. At any one point in time, a wide variety of behaviors are possible, some of which will be more adaptive than others for the current challenge.

Stable adaptive response behaviors are those that individuals frequently use when experiencing extreme difficulty and stress while attempting to respond to occupational challenges. Stable behaviors are characterized as hyperstable or rigid on the dysadaptive side of the continuum in that they present as a kind of "stuckness." They occur in all person factors (values, beliefs, movement, processing, and interacting). On the other side of the continuum, stable behaviors can simply be those habitual behaviors that we frequently perform with secondary energy, almost as if on autopilot. Habits exist when a pattern of behavior is consistently adaptive, efficiently and effectively serving our purposes well, and freeing our attention to other matters. However, sometimes circumstances change, and habits need to be adjusted. A response might be characterized as dysadaptive when a person rigidly sticks with an established habitual behavior even when the outcome is no longer efficient, effective, or satisfying.

It is important to recognize stable behaviors as "normal," even adaptive, when the individual feels overwhelmed by a particular challenge. Thus, their occurrence should be expected and not considered dysfunctional when they are used as a temporary balance-restoring mechanism. When hyperstability is used ineffectively for a protracted period, adaptation is hindered (Dallman et al., 2019). The story of The Graduate Student (Story 4-1) relates to the use of existing adaptive response modes and hyperstable behavior as a default (or first line of response) to a novel environmental demand.

One way that an occupational therapist guided by occupational adaptation constructs may intervene when someone is "stuck" is to recommend or help the person "break set," or interrupt the cycle in which they are stuck. In Figures 4-2 and 4-3, you might relate to the phenomenon that we sometimes get great ideas when doing mundane tasks, such as showering, driving, or walking about.

Mobile adaptive response behaviors, in contrast to stable behaviors, characterize the transition away from rigid habitual behaviors. Mobility can begin with flexibility, trying to do something differently. Like stable behaviors, mobile behaviors occur holistically and might involve patterns of movement, processing, and interacting. Mobile behaviors may follow stable behaviors as a transition to get the individual

CASE 4-2

The Researcher

Dr. Mensah was a 33-year-old physician from Ghana, Africa, who had come to the United States to study for a PhD in anatomy. As the result of an automobile accident, his nondominant left arm had to be amputated at the shoulder. His greatest concern was that he would be unable to complete the research for his dissertation, which involved the study of human brain tissue. After learning from Dr. Mensah what the external and internal role expectations were, the therapist—in collaboration with Dr. Mensah—developed a plan of intervention. They concluded that the most pressing need was to be able to continue the tasks associated with data collection (i.e., analysis and written reporting). To engage in the tasks of his chosen role, it was essential that Dr. Mensah develop new or modified adaptive response modes using one-handed approaches to respond to his occupational challenges until a prosthesis could be fitted and training in its use completed.

As part of his occupational adaptation intervention program, the therapist included occupational readiness goals, such as an increase in right upper extremity endurance, increased knowledge of assistive equipment and one-handed techniques, and fluidotherapy for pain in the right hand. His occupational activities included discussion and demonstration of his ability to carry out functions in his research laboratory (i.e., operation of a cryostat to prepare very thin slices of tissue samples for examination under a microscope). Dr. Mensah and the therapist made a trip to his laboratory to problem solve ways in which he could use one hand. Because Dr. Mensah was also interested in activities of daily living (ADLs) and instrumental ADLs, the intervention plan included his one-handed construction and the use of an assistive fingernail clipper and file board; ADL skills in dressing with assistive devices or one-handed techniques; driver re-education with the use of a spinner knob; and community activity, including filling a car with gasoline and asking for help when needed.

On a return trip to the clinic after discharge, Dr. Mensah reported to the therapist that he had installed a turning knob on the steering wheel of his car to allow him to drive with one hand. Dr. Mensah's preaccident existing adaptive response mode of using two hands could not successfully be used until his prosthesis was ready. He had to develop a new one-handed mode, which he used successfully. Thus, the therapist assisted Dr. Mensah in developing a new adaptive response mode. In the future when the prosthesis becomes a part of his functional picture, he will have to modify his previous two-handed and one-handed modes to accommodate to the prosthesis. He will likely continue the use of his new one-handed mode for certain tasks if he experiences the prosthesis to be cumbersome.

Case contributed by DeLana Honaker, PhD, OTR

"unstuck." Perhaps you baked a dozen cookies prepared from scratch, only to find them too flat and a little burnt. A mobile response might look like modifying your recipe for each of the next batches before putting them in the oven; instead of following the recipe (stability), you are trying other solutions (mobility). The mobile behaviors provide variability in solution attempts (a trial-and-error approach), some of which may provide adaptive movement or even a solution. Mobile behaviors can become hypermobile (i.e., highly variable, not well modulated, very active, often random, and without clear goal direction). In the example provided previously, a person might demonstrate hypermobility if every time they bake cookies, they disregard the recipe and add ingredients based on a whim. Mobility frequently functions as an intermediate step between hyperstable behaviors and a more adaptive blended approach, although this is not always the case. Eventually, we hope to see a transition to more systematic experimental behaviors, which lean into the blended behaviors that are described next. Let us look at Figure 4-3, which illustrates the case of the snappy dresser.

Chris had habits and routines that worked very well for them until the environment presented an unexpected demand. Their preferred outfit was unavailable, creating a press for mastery to maintain their identity as a "snappy dresser." Stable patterns of behavior did not solve the problem. The beginnings of mobility were tentative when trying to mend the damaged shirt, but when this did not work, a flurry of random and chaotic (hypermobile) behaviors followed. Out of this extreme and frantic behavior, a solution emerged! Chris discovered a new look that they were very pleased with. Although not efficient, the result was very effective and highly satisfying. This leads us to the third group of adaptive response behaviors.

Story and analysis contributed by Kyle Karen, MS, PhD

STORY 4-1

The Graduate Student

Brook was a first-year graduate student with an educational accommodation of extra time on tests and quizzes. Her challenge was to choose between taking examinations in traditional paper format or electronically (online), a choice offered to all the students in her cohort.

For the midterm assessment, 21 of the 28 students in her class opted for the online testing format. Of the seven students who opted for paper and pencil, four of them transferred their answers from paper to the online format to immediately receive their grades. Obtaining the grade immediately was a compelling benefit. Furthermore, taking the test electronically increased their comfort level with online assessment in anticipation of a future certification examination.

Brook, however, displayed increased anxiety over taking the test in an online format. She knew the benefits of the electronic format and conceded that she did need to "get used to taking tests on the computer." Yet, her reluctance to do so was so pronounced she declined to even transfer her answers from paper to the online form. Brook appeared to be hyperstabilized, unable to move away from familiar patterns of engagement in this occupation (test taking) even when there were clear benefits and a supportive environment (i.e., extended time, the option to transfer answers from her paper copy of the test, encouragement from her professor). She stated, "It just makes me nervous. I might get confused."

What is interesting about Brook's response is that she was a computer user and had been for many years. However, it was not novel technology that presented a problem for her; it was the novel use of technology that presented a challenge. She was not accustomed to testing in an online format. In addition, as a student receiving testing accommodations, she was accustomed to having the option for paper-and-pencil versions of tests throughout her academic career.

ANALYSIS

Humans are comfortable with the familiar. Change provokes anxiety. Individuals are sensitive to change based on context and client factors. For most students, a midterm examination provokes some degree of anxiety. For a student with learning differences, a midterm examination may provoke a heightened anxiety response proportionate to the perception of the challenge or threat. A change in the method of test delivery represents a change in the environmental demand associated with the role of the student. The resulting press for mastery requires an adaptive response on the part of the student.

Brook's pattern of a rigid, hyperstabilized response to an environmental demand created by a different use of technology was strongly influenced by her accumulated life experiences. Her skepticism may be the result of a press for mastery that is inconsistent with her deeply held beliefs about her capabilities.

Blended adaptive response behaviors are those exemplified by an efficient, effective, and satisfying balance of mobility and stability. Blended behaviors are modulated, goal directed, logical or insightful, and solution oriented. Blended behaviors range from the flexibility of mobile behaviors to the balance that leads to stability (Figure 4-4). It is important to remember that blended behaviors may not be the first behaviors seen in an attempt to respond adaptively and masterfully. The individual may use stable and/or mobile behaviors, perhaps moving in and out of these before arriving at a blended behavioral response. When the individual uses blended behaviors to find a truly adaptive response to one challenge, there is no assurance that blended behaviors will be used at the onset of a new challenge. All three types of behavior remain in our adaptation repertoire. In route to an

adaptive solution, we may use all three types of response behaviors at various times in situations in which the challenge is complex and multifaceted. Thus, the emergence of these behaviors is to be expected and not a cause for discouragement. Only if no adaptation develops after a reasonable period are stable and mobile variations considered dysadaptive.

The case of The Chess Player (Case 4-3) exhibits how the therapist facilitates adaptive movement through the various types of adaptive response behaviors. It is also an outstanding example of a therapist approaching treatment holistically. Instead of ignoring the patient's psychosocial dysfunction, the therapist attended to it therapeutically and effectively, thereby achieving the desired goals associated with the patient's physical dysfunction.

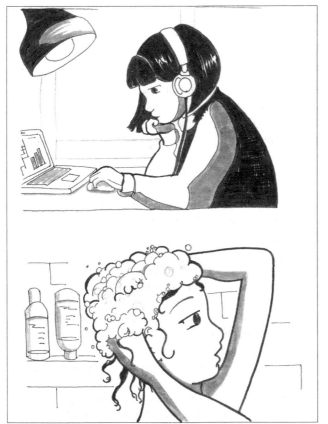

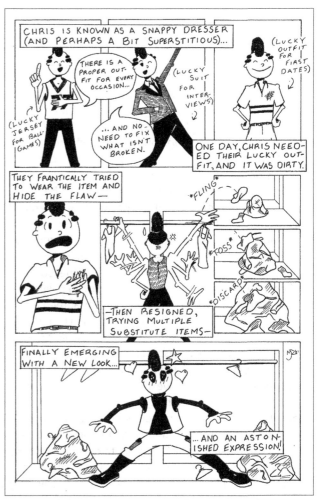

Figure 4-2. (Top) Kim worked on a school-related project for days and could not find a solution. (Bottom) While taking a shower after a long day at the computer, Kim had an enlightened insight that might solve the problem for the school project. (Illustrated by David Baxter.)

Figure 4-3. The snappy dresser. (Illustrated by Mitchell Reid.)

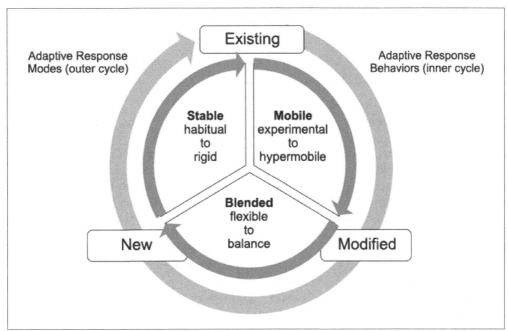

Figure 4-4. Cyclic representation of the adaptive response mechanism involving both adaptive response modes and adaptive response behaviors.

CASE 4-3

The Chess Player

Mr. Barnes was a 58-year-old man hospitalized for rehabilitation after a total hip replacement. He had a history of depression and presented with many behaviors consistent with obsessive-compulsive disorder. He was well-known for his chess-playing skill, as evidenced by his picture on the cover of a chess magazine. Mr. Barnes was extremely anxious and had difficulty focusing on therapy because of anxieties regarding such things as cleanliness, bowel movements, staff who were uncooperative to his many demands, medical bills, and so on.

In occupational therapy sessions, Mr. Barnes focused on complaints and anxieties, which his therapist and psychologist believed were more related to his fears regarding loss of control and death. In accordance with the physician's referral and the protocol for rehabilitation after total hip replacement, the therapist focused on educating Mr. Barnes about hip precautions. However, his anxieties interfered with his compliance with hip precautions. Mr. Barnes was hyperstable in his focus on anxiety and despair.

The therapist discussed with Mr. Barnes his feeling of loss of control and the accompanying behaviors he demonstrated. Together, they looked at the positive and negative aspects of these behaviors and how they affected his performance and satisfaction in daily life. They spent some time on relaxation techniques to help him get "unstuck" from his hyperstability. They agreed that he would make a list of his concerns before the occupational therapy sessions. He and the therapist then discussed the list and which concerns he could do something about, what his options were, and what things he could let go. The psychologist helped to educate the staff regarding obsessive-compulsive disorder and how they might better interact with Mr. Barnes.

Mr. Barnes responded to the plan and began to perform ADLs in a way that was somewhat satisfying to him. However, he was impulsive and had to receive constant cuing by the therapist to pay attention to hip precautions and safety (his hyperstability had been replaced by hypermobility). The therapist pointed out that attention to detail and the ability to remember rules was what made him successful in playing chess. She recommended that he use this same approach in remembering and executing the hip precaution "rules."

His impulsivity in ADLs began to decrease, and he prided himself on remembering the hip precaution rules. He still required occasional cuing in novel situations to comply with the precautions. His interaction with staff improved for those staff members who were able to give Mr. Barnes choices. At discharge 2 weeks later, he was functioning with modified independence in ADLs. He demonstrated his ability to generalize hip precautions to novel activities. His basic obsessive approach still pervaded his life, but he did occasionally initiate relaxation techniques. His list of concerns in the hospital became minimal, and he began to realistically assess his options regarding those concerns without assistance. Mr. Barnes was demonstrating behavior that was an adaptive blend of mobility and stability.

Case contributed by Joanna Lipoma, MOT, OTR

The occupational adaptation process is most obvious during life transitions that impact occupational functioning. These transitions may be normative (e.g., a transition from spouse to parent or student to professional) or unanticipated (e.g., the shift from an able-bodied young adult to a young adult with a spinal cord injury). During major life transitions, the adaptation process is most at risk for disruption. A premorbid adaptation process that is dysfunctional or functioning marginally will be vulnerable to profound impact. The well-functioning adaptation process will be less vulnerable but will be challenged to the limits of its intact and healthy operation. During these life transitions, the various classes of the adaptive response behaviors—stable, mobile, and blended—will be most evident.

The adaptive response mechanism is an abstract description of how the adaptive response begins to develop. Two occupational therapists who specialize in the practice of hand dysfunction created a model of how you might see the adaptive response mechanism in a client. These two therapists reflected on the responses they had seen in their clients and found striking examples of how their clients demonstrated the aspects of this mechanism. This model (Table 4-1) provides a good summary of the adaptive response mechanism in practice. It demonstrates responses that clients frequently exhibit as they progress through the challenges accompanying the need for adaptation after injury, trauma, or illness.

TABLE 4-1 **Adaptive Response Mechanism Examples From Upper Extremity Outpatient Practice**	
ADAPTATION ENERGY	
Primary	Learning exercise and use of equipment, splints, and assistive devices during treatment sessions
Secondary	Incorporating exercises and positioning into a daily routine; reintegration of the hand into self-care, work, and leisure activities
ADAPTIVE RESPONSE MODES	
Existing	Use of currently available coping skills, cognitive skills, problem-solving approaches
Modified	Enhancement of coping skills; enhanced self-discipline for adherence to the program; change routine to allow for treatment time
New	Development of new coping skills; owning the injury and recovery process; structuring time and gaining outside support to make time and energy available for treatment
ADAPTIVE RESPONSE BEHAVIORS	
Stable	Fear of reinjury; unwillingness to return to previous tasks or roles (e.g., the patient sees their role as the passive "recipient" of the treatment process and may be a passive participant in a treatment plan)
Mobile	Preoccupation with details of the treatment program; search for more options that will help; search for advice from anyone and everyone (e.g., the patient brings in popular media reports of unusual or novel treatment ideas)
Blended	Sees the injury as an event to be dealt with; takes initiative in treatment planning and implementation (e.g., active participant in a cooperatively designed treatment process)

Note: Model contributed by Gail Blom, OTR, CHT, CLT, MA, and Kimberly Norton, MA, LOTR, CHT.

Summary

Up to this point, we have talked about how occupational adaptation views the person and the occupational environment. We have addressed the occupational challenge and role expectations from both the person and the occupational environment. Once the person encounters an occupational challenge and begins to develop a response, the adaptive response mechanism comes into play. The adaptive response mechanism is part of the internal process that occurs as a person develops a response to an occupational challenge. Because adaptation is seen as an internal human process, we do not refer to adaptive equipment; rather, assistive devices might help facilitate an adaptation strategy. Along the same logic, we do not talk about adaptive environments, but people can modify the environment to support a person who needs to adapt. It may seem silly to be so picky about vocabulary, but even subtle implications set up by our choice of words influence how we think when engaging in clinical reasoning. In order to be intentional when facilitating therapeutic interactions, we think the words that guide our thoughts and actions really do matter.

The internal adaptive response mechanisms have been examined in this chapter and illustrated by therapist-reported cases. The second part of adaptive response generation is the adaptation gestalt, which is the topic of the next chapter. The adaptation gestalt describes how the person holistically responds in every situation.

A Deeper Dive

Of course, nothing stays new for long. So, at what point does a new adaptive response become an existing response mode? Theoretically, it would be when the response can be carried out with secondary energy. For example, what if my normal route to work is blocked by construction and I need to find a different route to get there? Consulting Google Maps is in my adaptation repertoire as an existing adaptive response to not knowing which way to go, especially in unfamiliar territory, so I consult the global positioning system (GPS) for a new route. This is an existing response mode and a stable behavior; it has often worked for me in the past. Driving a car is not new; however, driving a new route may present an occupational challenge because of the novelty of going a different

Neuro Spotlight

Activity-Dependent Plasticity

In addition to the primary and secondary energy discussed in the text, the adaptive response is generated through a form of neuroplasticity known as *activity-dependent plasticity*. Activity-dependent plasticity is evident in the learning that occurs from personal experiences and participation in engaging activities. Activity-dependent plasticity arises from internal neural activity as opposed to external stimulations, such as transcutaneous brain stimulation or drug-induced neuroplasticity. The brain's ability to remodel itself forms the basis of the brain's capacity to retain memories, improve motor function, and enhance comprehension and speech, among other things. Subsequently, it is this ability to retain and form memories associated with neural plasticity that contributes to the functions individuals perform on a daily basis. Activity-dependent neural plasticity occurs as a series of events that begins with signaling of molecules (e.g., calcium, dopamine, and glutamate, among others) during increased neuronal activity. The molecular signals then initiate a cascade of neural events that ultimately results in changes in gene expression.

The brain's ability to adapt through participation in goal-directed activity allows us to gain relative mastery of skills. For example, an amateur musician will likely play the piano poorly, yet with continuous practice can learn the skill of piano playing. Furthermore, a person with a neurologic disorder such as a spinal cord injury or stroke can gain relative mastery over many skills, increasing function and participation through purposeful engagement in activities and practice.

Recommended Readings

Dunlop, S. A. (2008). Activity-dependent plasticity: Implications for recovery after spinal cord injury. *Trends in Neurosciences, 31*(8), 410-418. https://doi.org/10.1016/j.tins.2008.05.004

Tropea, D., Kreiman, G., Lyckman, A., Mukherjee, S., Yu, H., Hrong, S., & Sur, M. (2006). Gene expression changes and molecular pathways mediating activity-dependent plasticity in visual cortex. *Nature Neuroscience, 9,* 660-668. https://doi.org/10.1038/nn1689

way. If the GPS directions take me into a neighborhood I have not been before and down streets completely unfamiliar to me, I am likely to use more primary energy and modify my usual driving behaviors (e.g., put down my coffee cup, read all road signs, look for unexpected obstructions, and attend to the directions provided). If the construction takes several days or weeks, my "modified" response starts to feel normal because it now exists in my adaptive repertoire and working memory; I no longer have to consult GPS to make sure I take the correct route, and I can return to a more stable response mode while driving to work. What is a daily routine that if interrupted would cause you to alter your response? How long would it take for a modified or new response to feel normal?

Take-Away Messages

◊ Existing, modified, and new adaptive response modes all have the potential to be adaptive or dysadaptive depending on the specifics of the occupational challenge at hand.

◊ Stable, mobile, and blended adaptive response behaviors are all potentially adaptive yet can also lead to dysadaptive responses depending on the prevailing circumstances (context).

◊ Existing adaptive response modes are those that have been deemed successful and integrated into a person's adaptation repertoire.

◊ Both primary and secondary adaptation energy are available for addressing occupational challenges. When primary energy is ineffective in producing satisfying responses, secondary energy is an efficient mechanism to fuel creative problem solving.

References

Carlson, R. (1997). *Don't sweat the small stuff … and it's all small stuff*. Hyperion.

Dallman, A., Boyd, B., & Harrop, C. (2019). The role of occupational inflexibility in down syndrome [Abstract]. *Seventh Annual Proceedings of The Society for the Study of Occupation: USA* (pp. 43-45). https://www.sso-usa.net/assets/docs/proceedings_2019.pdf

Dolecheck, J. R., & Schkade, J. K. (1999). The extent dynamic standing endurance is effected when CVA subjects perform personally meaningful activities rather than nonmeaningful tasks. *Occupational Therapy Journal of Research, 19*(1), 40-53. https://doi.org/10.1177/153944929901900103

Garber, S. L. (2016). The prepared mind, 2016 Eleanor Clarke Slagle lecture. *American Journal of Occupational Therapy, 70,* 7006150010. https://doi.org/10.5014/ajot.2016.706001

Gilfoyle, E., Grady, A., & Moore, J. (1990). *Children adapt.* (2nd ed.). SLACK Incorporated.

Guest, E. A. (n.d.). It couldn't be done. *Poetry Foundation.* https://www.poetryfoundation.org/poems/44314/it-couldnt-be-done

Ramón y Cajal, S. (1999). *Advice for a young investigator* (N. Swanson & L. W. Swanson, Trans., 2nd ed.). MIT Press.

Schultz, S., & Schkade, J. K. (1997). Adaptation. In C. Christiansen & C. Baum (Eds.), *Occupational therapy: Enabling function and well-being* (2nd ed.). SLACK Incorporated.

Selye, H. (1956). *The stress of life.* McGraw-Hill.

Try It On

Now let's dig a little deeper. Reflect on how you went about preparing to respond to your occupational challenge. The following tables will help lead you through the process.

Occupational Challenge (from Chapter 3): _____

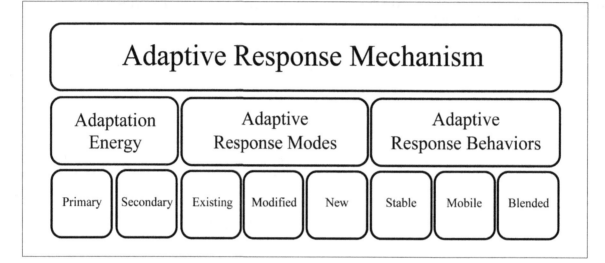

Let's enlarge each of these components for a closer look. Remember we are continuing to focus on your identified occupational challenge.

ADAPTATION ENERGY	YES/NO
Primary While engaged in responding to your particular challenge, did you find yourself initially focused with high energy and high concentration to your task and remain there for the duration of the activity?	
Secondary While engaged in responding to your particular challenge, did you find yourself at first highly focused and concentrating on your task, then leaving it for a time to do something else? Did you then return to your task and find you had made progress on a problem solution even while actively doing something else?	
Further observations:	

(continued)

ADAPTIVE RESPONSE MODES	YES/NO
Existing Did you find that you engaged with your challenge the same way that you always have? Routine? "Same old, same old?"	
Modified Did you find that you were engaged with your challenge in some ways the same, but you also tried something different? "Living slightly on the edge?"	
New Did you find that you approached your challenge with a whole different approach? "Life in the fast lane?"	
Other thoughts:	

ADAPTIVE RESPONSE BEHAVIORS	YES/NO
Stable Did you find that when you were engaged in responding to your challenge, you were trying what had worked in the past? Sticking to a plan? Or just plain stuck (hyperstable)?	
Mobile Did you find that when you were engaged in responding to your challenge, you were switching gears? Using trial and error? Or moving fast and in no apparent planned and organized direction (hypermobile)?	
Blended Did you find that when you were engaged in responding to your challenge, you experienced thoughtful problem solving and adaptation based on a combination of reason and creativity (blended mobility and stability)?	

(continued)

When you were preparing your responses, did you find yourself "bouncing around" among these three types of behavior? If you did, that's okay. Remember these are simply classes of behavior, all of which exist to help with an adaptive response.

Additional Reflections:

In the occupational adaptation process, these components (adaptation energy, adaptive response modes, and adaptive response behaviors) are dynamic actions, flowing naturally in the context of the challenge. In the next chapter, we examine the adaptation gestalt or plan of action.

CHAPTER 5

Adaptation Gestalt
What's the Plan to Carry Out the Response?

*Thus every matter, if it is to be done well,
calls for the attention of the whole person.*
—Martin Luther

Chapter 4 described the adaptive response mechanisms (i.e., adaptation energy, modes, behaviors) that are essential to adaptive response generation. The remaining component of adaptive response generation is the adaptation gestalt. A gestalt represents the idea that the whole is greater than the sum of its parts. The adaptation gestalt is a way to think about holistic responding and intervention. The adaptation gestalt supports or inhibits the work of the adaptive response mechanism (adaptation energy, adaptive response modes, and adaptive response behaviors), and simultaneously (and instantaneously), configures a holistic response to every challenge. When the response is not holistic, it is not likely to be fully efficient, effective, and satisfying.

The Adaptation Gestalt

An important assumption of occupational adaptation is that people holistically engage in occupations with all aspects of their person system (Figure 5-1) present and interacting to support performance skills (motor, process, and interaction skills) needed for every response. Based on dominant factors, all skills then must be configured to effectively produce an occupational response. In occupational adaptation, we refer to this holistic approach as the *adaptation gestalt*.

Evetts, C. L., & Baxter, M. F. *Cases and Concepts in Occupational Adaptation:
Translating Theory into Action* (pp. 47-56).
DOI: 10.4324/9781003522850-5

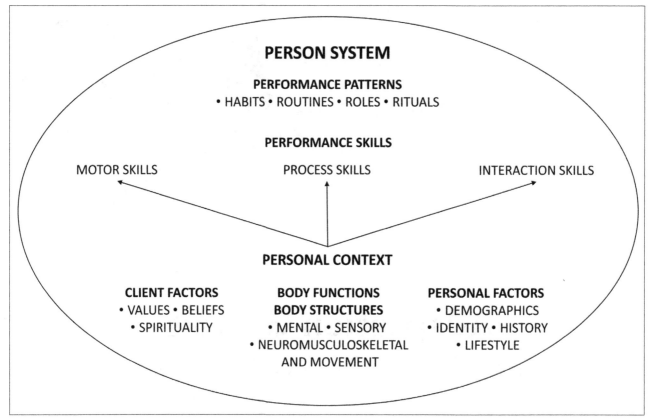

Figure 5-1. Holistic engagement in occupations requires the entire person system working in concert.

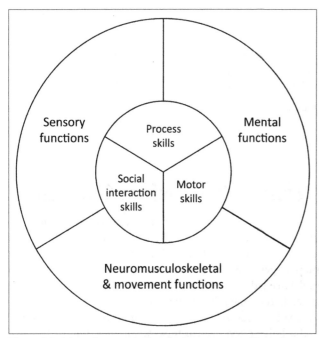

Figure 5-2. Adaptation gestalt. *Note:* Body structures and body functions (sensory, mental, neuromusculoskeletal and movement functions) are all present to support the performance skills needed to respond adaptively to an occupational challenge.

Although all person system elements are present in a holistic response, each element is not necessarily present to the same degree in every adaptation gestalt. See Figure 5-2 for a generic adaptation gestalt configuration. The pie chart in the center represents the relative balance of performance skills being applied to a task. Of course, these skills are dependent on body functions being at the ready. The elements in this double pie chart are not meant to align specific body functions with certain skill sets; remember that gestalt refers to the whole being more significant than individual parts. A well-functioning adaptation gestalt is dependent on the holistic configuration of available body functions to support a holistic array of performance skills to address an occupational challenge. Obviously, all of this occurs within a larger context, but we deal with that later.

The specific performance skills (center) needed to address an occupational challenge can only emerge if the body functions are balanced to support the task. Body functions need to be available to different degrees based on the demands of a specific task. For a predominantly motor task such as running, the neuromusculoskeletal and movement functions need to be fully engaged to provide the foundation for reciprocal movement of the lower extremities. To a lesser degree, but nevertheless important, are sensory functions that support running. Proprioception, vestibular, and visual

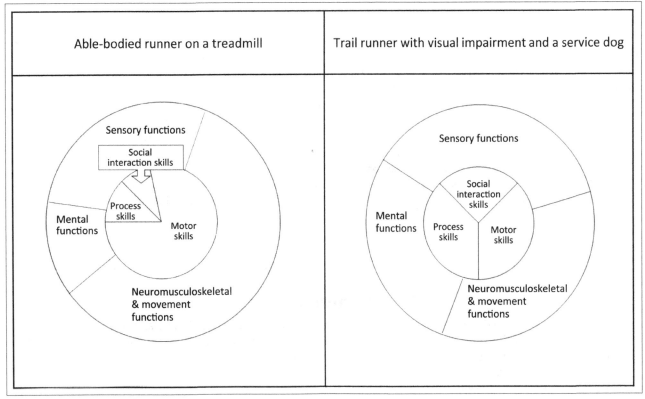

Figure 5-3. Adaptation gestalts: running.

sensing contribute to balance to avoid tipping over and to recover from stumbling when obstacles are encountered. Mental functions, although needed for awareness of one's surroundings, may be minimized as less active. Of course, these are general assumptions and may only apply to an able body running on a treadmill. A different configuration will be appropriate for a person with significant visual impairment (sensory function) who is running on a park trail with their service dog. They may rely more on sensory functions, such as hearing, touch, and smell, to increase awareness of their surroundings, and they may require greater use of mental functions to support processing their sensory data and communicating with their dog and other runners encountered on the trail. Figure 5-3 illustrates the possible differences in adaptation gestalt for these two runners. Based on these hypothetical adaptation gestalt configurations, which one do you suspect might have longer endurance? Assuming each has a comparable cardiovascular system, what might influence how long each may endure the run? (Hint: Remember to consider the adaptation gestalt in relationship to all aspects of the adaptive response mechanisms [i.e., adaptation energy, modes, behaviors].)

We can take this example even further. Consider the broader context and resulting adaptation gestalt configuration for a runner whose cultural expectations dictate clothing or one who has a strong history related to running or not running or whether habitual behaviors support or interfere with the act of running. There are infinite possibilities for adaptation gestalts to be efficient, effective, and satisfying or dysadaptive in some way depending on both personal and environmental contexts.

Different tasks require different adaptation gestalt configurations. If a task is essentially problem solving, then the specific mental functions supporting one's gestalt should be intact so that processing skills are dominant and supported by thinking and reasoning while providing an adaptive level of motivation and keeping factors such as anxiety from interfering with performance. At the same time, the movement-related functions should be operating to provide physical mobility or stability appropriately, and the sensory functions should be operating to support a modulated response to stimuli. A student taking an examination probably needs the plan just described.

When the task primarily demands communication/interaction skills, as in comforting a friend who has lost a family member, the mental functions must be most sensitive and effective, with process skills appropriately involved to assist with empathic reasoning. At the same time, the movement-related and sensory functions will be ready to support an activity that will allow the friend to carry out the comforting actions adaptively.

In other words, the adaptation gestalt balance will differ from one situation to another if adaptive occupational functioning is to be realized. There is no one "balanced" adaptation gestalt that fits all persons and situations. It is highly idiosyncratic to the situation and the individual. The case of The Alarmed Student (Case 5-1) illustrates how the adaptation gestalt works by examining a dysadaptive response to an unexpected sensory interruption.

It is important when developing a therapeutic intervention to recognize that all of a person's body functions and performance skills are engaged in each occupational response. When the occupational adaptation process has become dysfunctional because of trauma, disease, chronic conditions, or other factors, the process cannot be improved without attention to the whole person regardless of the nature of the disabling condition. For example, if an individual is so depressed after suffering a stroke that they have no desire to participate in rehabilitation, the therapist will be hard-pressed to achieve any therapeutic results in communication, motor, or processing skills while their emotional response is dominating the adaptation gestalt. If the therapist can facilitate a change in the adaptation gestalt to bring the body functions into a better balance for the task of rehabilitation, the impact of therapy will be much more effective in addressing the patient's occupational adaptation process. When the person is adaptive, they will build functional skills.

CASE 5-1

The Alarmed Student

Brian is an 18-year-old student who has autism and is nonverbal. One day, Brian was alone in the hallway of his high school on his way to the bathroom when a fellow student ran past him, accidentally hitting and triggering the fire alarm with his backpack. A high-pitched beeping began with flashing lights, and the sudden loud slamming of the fire doors started Brian's escalation. It is unusual for Brian to be in the hallway during a fire alarm. Generally, the staff notifies him beforehand to reduce the possibility of an escalation. Although he has participated in fire drills before, it was a new experience to be near the alarm and to not have his typical warning and staff support. There was no time for staff to intervene; they were as surprised by the alarm as he had been.

At the start of his escalation, Brian began to screech loudly. The hallway began to fill with high schoolers racing loudly through the hallways, bumping into him in their hurry to evacuate. He screamed and pounded on the walls, windows, and doors, yelling and striking out against anyone attempting to help him out of the building. No longer surprised by the alarm and unable to "flee," he was now in "fight" mode and began to attack both students and staff (scratching, punching, and kicking). The staff tried to remind him of where he could go to escape the noise, but he did not heed their instructions. When the hallways were finally empty, staff could escort him to his designated safe spot, but he remained upset for hours.

After several hours, Brian was able to return to class, and he was responding to directions. With prompting, he took deep breaths and counted to five before entering the classroom. However, his return to class was short-lived because he was unable to "keep it together," and he was escorted home earlier than hoped.

ANALYSIS

At the start of the escalation, Brian's sensory functions were flooded, and his adaptive response was dependent on a highly emotional response (mental function). His adaptation gestalt was dominated by the specific mental function of emotion. His processing skills were so diminished in the situation that staff intervention was unable to help him access memory or reasoning to identify helpful strategies. As the hallway filled with people, his emotional state and inability to access problem-solving strategies gave way, and his adaptation gestalt focus shifted to his global mental functions and the primitive urge to fight his way out. Throughout this situation, Brian's processing skills remained small and unused. He was eventually able to return to class as his adaptation gestalt shifted to allow his mental and sensory functions to be primary, and his motor reactions (driven by dominant neuromusculoskeletal and movement functions) were no longer overactive. However, he was unable to maintain a balanced adaptation gestalt appropriate for the classroom, and he needed a shift in his occupational environment to recover, so he was sent home.

Case and analysis contributed by Teri K. Rupp, PhD, OTR/L, C/NDT

Focusing on an occupation that is important to the client is the optimal way to facilitate an adaptation gestalt configuration that is most likely to produce an improvement in occupational functioning. The case of The Husband Caregiver (Case 5-2) illustrates how the therapist facilitated a rebalancing of the adaptation gestalt to produce a therapeutic outcome based on the demands of the client's primary occupational role.

The adaptation gestalt is a simple, straightforward way to conceptualize how an individual holistically engages in an occupational response. This way of creating an image of one's response may be useful in assisting individuals to anticipate the outcome of their occupational response before the response has been acted out, and thus, provide one way to self-correct dysfunctional responses. The case of The Newlywed (Case 5-3) illustrates how shifting the focus of intervention helped to create a reconfiguration of the adaptation gestalt for a young woman undergoing cancer treatment.

CASE 5-2

The Husband Caregiver

Mr. Brown was an 82-year-old man who was hospitalized after a stroke. His previous medical history included hypertension and prostate cancer. His wife of 54 years was expected to live no more than 6 months because of terminal lung cancer. Several years earlier she had been diagnosed with breast cancer, which was followed by a mastectomy. She had never regained full range of motion or strength in her affected extremity. As a result of Mrs. Brown's challenges, Mr. Brown had been assisting her with upper extremity dressing, self-care, and cooking for many years. In the initial assessment, when the therapist asked Mr. Brown about his primary occupational interest, he indicated that it was to do everything he could to help his wife in the ways to which they had become accustomed (his role as her caregiver). An assessment of Mr. Brown's person systems revealed the following:

- Neuromusculoskeletal and motor functions: Active range of motion in the left extremity was within functional limits with muscle strength and grip strength rated as a 3+ out of 5, and limited range of motion in the right extremity with muscle and grip strength rated as a 2+ out of 5. He required minimum assistance in bed mobility. His static sitting balance was rated as good, whereas his dynamic sitting balance was rated as fair+. His endurance was sufficient to tolerate sitting on the side of the bed with minimum fatigue during an evaluation that lasted approximately 45 minutes.

- Sensory functions: Bilaterally, his sensation (light touch, pain, stereognosis, kinesthesia, proprioception, and temperature) was within functional limits.

- Mental functions: Mr. Brown was oriented to person, place, and date. His attention span and concentration during the evaluation were within functional limits. The assessment revealed a husband who was depressed and tearful as he discussed with the therapist his wife's impending death. He expressed guilt that his prostate cancer had been healed while his wife's cancer had not. He voiced a strong desire to concentrate only on spending time with his wife. He was not interested in therapy for himself.

- Occupational environment: The couple lived in a two-bedroom home with assistive bathroom equipment that included a tub transfer bench, an elevated toilet seat, and a handheld shower. The Browns lived in a neighborhood where the neighbors were supportive.

Mr. Brown's occupational role of caregiver became the basis for intervention. It was clear to the therapist that Mr. Brown's adaptation gestalt was dominated by emotions (mental functions) because he was depressed and grieving, making it difficult to engage motor and processing skills, which were the reasons for the occupational therapy referral. The therapist's task was to develop an intervention that would facilitate the reconfiguration of Mr. Brown's adaptation gestalt to reflect the importance of the mental functions at this time in his life while also allowing the sensory and neuromusculoskeletal and movement functions to become more active.

(continued)

The therapist devised all aspects of the intervention plan with Mr. Brown's preferred occupational role of caregiver directing her thinking. She developed occupational readiness interventions (interventions in the body functions to help prepare for the occupation of caregiver). These interventions included the following:

- Minimal resistance Theraband activities and balloon batting activities with his wife; wrist weights were added as tolerated
- Medium resistance hand putty exercise and proprioceptive neuromuscular facilitation trunk stabilization exercise
- Simple hygiene and hemidressing techniques for himself

Occupational activities (intervention in which the client was actively engaged in his chosen occupational role) included the following:

- Assisting his wife with upper extremity dressing using assistive devices
  - To address endurance, dynamic sitting balance, trunk stabilization, upper extremity strength, grip strength, hemidressing technique, and motor planning
- Assisting her with simple hygiene using his affected right arm as a stabilizing unit
  - To address weight-bearing, proprioception, balance, and upper extremity strength
- Working with her to put together a photo album
  - To address processing and communication/interaction skills and mental functions as stories were retold with dates/places/people
  - To address movement functions and motor skills with grip strength and endurance
  - Mental functions and processing skills for the grief process
- Cooking easy breakfasts/lunches/dinners with her
  - To address holistic engagement in everyday living

Case based on Ross (1994)

CASE 5-3

The Newlywed

Mandy was a 31-year-old female newlywed who presented to the emergency department with sudden-onset paralysis in her bilateral lower extremities. Upon further diagnostic workup, she was diagnosed with multiple myeloma, which had led to a tumor pressing on her spinal cord, impairing motor function to her legs and feet. In addition to central nervous system impairment, the patient had peripheral damage to her left hand and arm due to a tumor on her humerus, which was previously dismissed as a blood clot. She developed hypersensitivity in her left hand, held her arm in a guarded posture, and demonstrated significant upper extremity functional limitations due to motor and sensory impairment.

Mandy had previously been employed as a child life specialist. She thrived in her helping role as she brought child-friendly play to the hospital for children with cancer. Mandy's diagnosis forced her to take a medical leave of absence, and she was unsure if she would ever return to her role at work. At the time of diagnosis, Mandy had been married to her husband for merely 6 months and was still adjusting to her new role as a wife. Mandy enjoyed shopping and throwing parties with friends, and she placed a high value on her physical appearance.

Over 3 weeks, Mandy was thrown into cancer treatment and occupational and physical therapies in acute care at the hospital followed by inpatient rehabilitation admission. Initially, the occupational therapist wrote goals primarily addressing sensorimotor deficits given the patient's physical limitations, including transfers, mobility, self-care, and work. Despite the importance of regaining independence, mobility, and the use of her left upper extremity for self-care tasks, Mandy experienced significant psychosocial disruption. Mandy's mood, affect, and engagement changed because of the numerous losses she experienced—her job, role as wife at home, party hostess, and physical identity with the new knowledge she would lose her hair and require a wheelchair to get around.

(continued)

In this case, the adaptation gestalt demonstrated an overwhelming dominance in the mental functions. Despite the importance of targeting deficit areas in the sensory and motor functions, Mandy was focused on the social ramifications of her diagnosis and was unable to move forward. As the occupational therapist picked up on these cues and Mandy's lack of motivation, she began to incorporate activities to tap into her altruistic, friendly personality. Mandy started to bake her favorite recipes from home, including her famous chocolate chip banana bread, and shared with others in the hospital, which gave her a sense of purpose and pride. She helped welcome other patients to the unit during the daily breakfast gatherings, showing them around the unit and introducing them to other staff and patients. Through these experiences, Mandy was motivated to get out of bed, transfer between surfaces, and stand for baking and washing dishes in the kitchen. The occupational therapist eventually began a conversation about home modifications and introduced alternative strategies to perform home management and self-care tasks, such as laundry and bathing. Over time, in collaboration between the patient and the therapist, a more effective adaptation gestalt configuration was achieved, and Mandy was able to reach a more appropriate balance among all elements of her person system and progress in rehabilitation.

Case contributed by Emily M. Rich, MOT, OTR/L

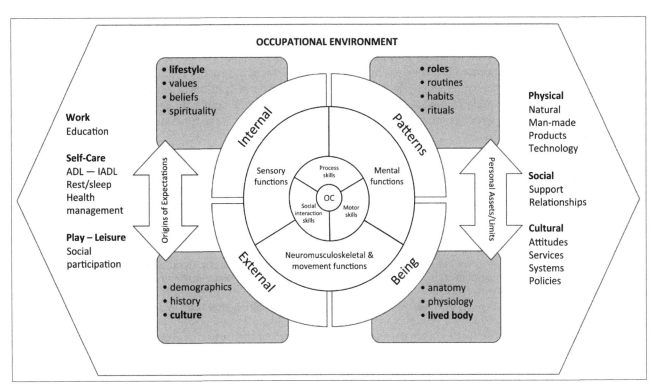

Figure 5-4. Occupational challenge in context.

As previously stated, the adaptation gestalt is dependent on the full context of an occupational challenge, including both personal and environmental contexts and their related expectations. Let us look at Figure 5-4 for an occupational challenge in full context.

Figure 5-4 is a configuration of the context of an occupation (center) in which performance skills emerge (small pie) as a result of relative balance in body functions (middle pie). Recall that these two pie charts are ever-changing to find an effective adaptation gestalt configuration. All of this is influenced by personal context (outer ring) as experienced in the context of the larger occupational environment (hexagon). Seeing a concrete representation of all that surrounds an occupational challenge is a reminder of the importance of the desire, demand, and press for mastery. The challenge for the therapist is to identify the person's desire and adjust the environment's demands to create an enticing press for mastery in the form of a just-right occupational challenge. Without press, no adaptation process can proceed.

NEURO SPOTLIGHT

Adaptive Plasticity

The neural system contributes to the adaptive response through its ability to adjust and change. This neural plasticity is also referred to as *adaptive plasticity*. Adaptive plasticity encompasses the changes seen in the brain's neural function and structure, which enables the brain to adjust in response to experiences, contributes to compensation for loss of movement, and maximizes remaining functions in the event of brain injury. Neurophysiologic, neuroanatomic, and neuroimaging studies conducted over the past 4 decades illustrate that the cerebral cortex is dynamic, changing both functionally and structurally over time. There is evidence of brain remapping of functions seen on neuroimaging studies with clients who are post–cerebrovascular accident and who engage in intense, structured, and function-based rehabilitation of the upper extremity (Taub et al., 2014). Additionally, cortical reorganization is known to be accompanied by changes in dendritic and synaptic structures and alterations in the regulation of neurotransmitter processing. Differences in connectivity are also observed using neuroimaging of different parts of the brain resulting from learning as seen in comparing expert musicians to novice musicians (Gaser & Schlaug, 2003).

Changes in the neural structures and processes can be adaptive or maladaptive. Adaptive changes due to neuroplasticity occur when the outcome is an improvement, such as a functional gain (Cohen et al., 1997). Maladaptive changes are noted when negative outcomes occur, such as injury or loss of function. An example of maladaptive plasticity in humans is focal dystonia in which impairment in sensory motor function occurs as the result of excessive repetitive movements, which is often seen in musician's dystonia or writer's cramp (Quartarone et al., 2006). Another example of maladaptation is the gradual increased spasticity seen with a person post–cerebrovascular accident who has little rehabilitation or motivation to increase function and movement in the affected extremity.

RECOMMENDED READINGS

Cohen, L. G., Celnik, P., Pascual-Leone, A., Corwell, B., Falz, L., Dambrosia, J., Honda, M., Sadato, N., Gerloff, C, Catalá, M. D., & Hallett, M. (1997). Functional relevance of cross-modal plasticity in blind humans. *Nature, 389*(6647), 180-183. https://doi.org/10.1038/38278

Gaser, C., & Schlaug, G. (2003). Brain structures differ between musicians and non-musicians. *The Journal of Neuroscience, 23*(27), 9240-9245. https://doi.org/10.1523/JNEUROSCI.23-27-09240.2003

Mark, V., & Taub, E. (2017). Constraint-induced movement therapy for chronic hemiparesis: Neuroscience evidence from basic laboratory research and quantitative structural brain MRI in patients with diverse disabling neurological disorders (S43.003). *Neurology, 88*(16 Supplement), S43.003.

Nudo, R. J. (2003). Adaptive plasticity in motor cortex: Implications for rehabilitation after brain injury. *Journal of Rehabilitation Medicine, Supplement, 41,* 7-10.

Nudo, R. J. (2007). The role of skill versus use in the recovery of motor function after stroke. *OTJR Occupation, Participation and Health, 27*(Suppl. 1), 24S-32S.

Quartarone, A., Siebner, H. R., & Rothwell, J. C. (2006). Task-specific hand dystonia: Can too much plasticity be bad for you? *Trends in Neurosciences, 29,* 192-199. https://doi.org/10.1016/j.tins.2006.02.007

Taub, E., Uswatte, G., & Mark, V. W. (2014). The functional significance of cortical reorganization and the parallel development of CI therapy. *Frontiers in Human Neuroscience, 8,* 396. https://doi.org/10.3389/fnhum.2014.00396

Let us return to the example at the beginning of this chapter—running. Imagine yourself with a challenge to run. What would fuel your desire for mastery? Getting to class on time? Trying to catch a bus? Rushing to remove a child from danger? Beating your personal best on a favorite running path? Once you have determined how to tap into the desire, demand, and press for mastery of an occupational challenge that involves running, consider all of the elements in Figure 5-4 to get the big picture of what may impact your performance. Which of these many factors is within your control to affect change? Which are imposed and feel constraining? Apply the same scenario to someone you know. Use empathy and reasoning to determine how you might intervene if their desire for mastery was impeded. What supports can be built upon? What challenges threaten success?

A Deeper Dive

In his 2017 Eleanor Clarke Slagle lecture, Dr. Roger Smith (2017) proposed a Metaphysical Physical–Emotive Theory of Occupation and described the need for persons to have a balanced approach to occupations.

> Many of our core occupation-based intervention strategies may have evolved out of this need to help balance these domains of reality. Think of the soldiers from the early 1900s receiving occupational therapy. They were set up with occupations to help structure feelings or, conversely, behaviors to provoke exploration and creativity. These are opposite strategies, but both were intended to balance a person with a skewed hyperactive emotiveness or physical reality, respectively. (p. 10)

Your occupational challenge (if your desire for mastery is strong) is to unpack this quote and align it with concepts of relative mastery. Imagine the soldier's adaptation gestalt as a result of trauma experienced in the war, and then consider how the occupational therapist used concepts of adaptation energy to facilitate adaptive response modes and behaviors.

TAKE-AWAY MESSAGES

◊ The concept of an adaptation gestalt is a way to visualize how a person's configuration of body functions can support or limit their ability to access or improve performance skills.

◊ A relative balance of mental, sensory, and neuromusculoskeletal and movement functions is needed if performance skills are to emerge.

◊ We (humans) bring our holistic selves to every occupational encounter and challenge; there is no adaptation in compartmentalization.

References

Ross, M. M. (1994, August 11). Applying theory to practice. *OT Week,* 16-17.

Smith, R. O. (2017). Technology and occupation: Past, present, and the next 100 years of theory and practice (Eleanor Clarke Slagle Lecture). *American Journal of Occupational Therapy, 71,* 7106150010. https://doi.org/10.5014/ajot.2017.716003

Try It On

Don't let the word gestalt deter you. This concept, as stated previously, is simply your "plan of action." For example, an occupational therapy fieldwork student enters their first patient's room with the task to begin an initial assessment. They find themself so nervous they cannot conceptualize how to begin the assessment. Their mind is inundated by the multitudes of assessments they have learned in school as they mentally scan through them with the hope that the right one will surface. They think about how disappointed their clinical instructor will be when they find that the assessment hasn't progressed. They widen their base of support, grasp their clipboard tightly, and try to ignore their shaking knees.

Been there? The following depicts how this student's gestalt may have looked. Notice that although their psychosocial system predominates, their cognitive and sensorimotor components are still present.

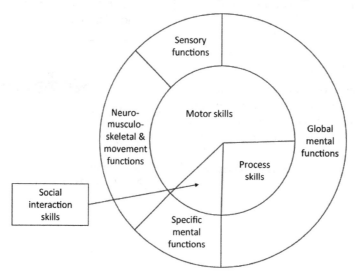

Now it's your turn. Consider the occupational challenge that you identified in Chapter 4. Take a look at your adaptation gestalt and how you generated your response. Using the circle as a pie, separate the person divisions and their involvement with your challenge.

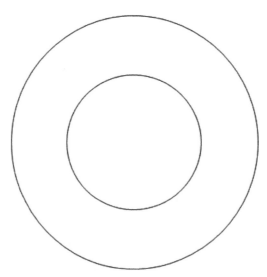

Any reflective thoughts?

You've finally responded to the challenge at hand. The next chapter explains how individuals go about evaluating the outcome of their attempts to respond adaptively and masterfully. This will involve a discussion of the next subprocess of the system—the adaptive response evaluation subprocess.

CHAPTER 6

Adaptive Response Evaluation, Relative Mastery

What's Going on Here?

I've failed over and over and over again in my life and that is why I succeed.
—*Michael Jordan*

*Learning and innovation go hand in hand. The arrogance of success is
to think that what you did yesterday will be sufficient for tomorrow.*
—*William Pollard*

Adaptive Response Evaluation

After the occupational response has been carried out, the next important step is for the individual to evaluate the outcome produced by the response. This evaluation takes place through the action of the adaptive response evaluation subprocess. For adaptation to occur, we must evaluate our occupational responses. Otherwise, we continue to repeat previous responses whether or not they were useful in achieving the intended goal. In other words, the leading edge of adaptation is awareness that the response needs to change for some perceived reason.

This self-evaluation process generally occurs on a subconscious level as we go about our normal daily routines. We behave and perform in ways that work for us based on experience and current levels of success, most often without having to think too much about it. However, when a problem occurs or an unexpected obstacle is presented, we are pressed to evaluate our response and adjust to remain adaptive and successful. When an individual gets stuck, usually because of a life transition or novel situation, it helps to bring that subliminal evaluation to a conscious level for an intentional shift to occur.

The self-evaluation process begins with activation of the evaluation function. One might initiate evaluation by asking themselves, "What's going on here?" Occupational adaptation

Evetts, C. L., & Baxter, M. F. *Cases and Concepts in Occupational Adaptation: Translating Theory into Action* (pp. 57-65).
DOI: 10.4324/9781003522850-6

proposes that the core action of the self-evaluation process is a phenomenological assessment called *relative mastery*. The word "phenomenological" emphasizes that relative mastery is an individualistic experience in evaluating the quality of an occupational response. Is relative mastery the same thing as skill mastery? Definitely not! We want to be clear about that. Do not confuse relative mastery with skill mastery, which is evaluated by an external source with external criteria to guide the evaluation.

Relative mastery consists of three properties:

1. Efficiency, which refers to the process (i.e., the use of time, energy, and resources)
2. Effectiveness, which refers to the product (i.e., the extent to which the response achieved the desired goal)
3. Satisfaction to self and others, which refers to the extent to which the person experiences satisfaction with the outcome and the extent to which relevant others indicate satisfaction with the outcome

Let us look at an example of a professional tennis player to illustrate the difference between relative mastery and skill mastery. Suppose we have a world-class tennis player. For 1 week they are playing in a major tournament where they are the top seed (officials who run the tournament expect them to win the tournament). They make it to the final match where they lose in three sets (the worst possible outcome). As they evaluate their performance in the tennis tournament, their self-assessment might look like the following:

- Efficiency: Because the match was relatively short, they used less time, energy, and personal resources than they would have if the match had been longer. Therefore, their efficiency was relatively high.
- Effectiveness: Not effective because they did not win.
- Satisfaction to self and others: Unsatisfying to the player and their fans, who wanted them to win; satisfying to those who wanted their opponent to win.

Suppose the next week the same tennis player is again playing in a major tournament. This time, they win in a grueling five-set match. They might evaluate their relative mastery as follows:

- Efficiency: Not efficient because it was a long match that took a great deal of time, energy, and personal resources.
- Effectiveness: Very effective because they won.
- Satisfaction to self and others: A very satisfying outcome; it is satisfying to win in a long, demanding match. Tennis-watching society also likes a five-set, demanding match.

The important point to be made here is that the skill mastery of the tennis player was the same over the 2 weeks; yet, their experience of relative mastery changed markedly from 1 week to the next. In the personal story of The Gymnast (Story 6-1), a new understanding of external expectations within the competitive context was key to reassessing relative mastery.

The gymnast was able to resolve her discontent by assessing relative mastery, realizing others were satisfied even though she was not, and shifting her role identity to achieve relative mastery. This adaptive response on her part has since generalized to her approach to her work, valuing the role of team member over a role that keeps her separated from others.

Similarly, the client with whom the therapist is intervening may have criteria that are important to them that do not show up on the therapist's assessment as an external evaluator. The therapist is likely using various assessment tools, such as standardized, norm-referenced, or functional independence evaluations. These externally determined evaluations are of merit for documentation and reimbursement purposes; however, from the standpoint of occupational adaptation, these evaluations are supplemented by the client's self-assessment of relative mastery. The client has a perspective of their internal expectations and the expectations of a specific environment on which intervention is focused. For example, the therapist may evaluate a skill competence level as low because of movement substitution patterns that deviate from an established norm. However, a client may view the same personal response as being reasonably efficient, very effective, and highly satisfying to self and others because the response is carried out in a manner that is consonant with internal expectations and physical, social, and cultural expectations of the relevant occupational environment. For example, therapists frequently report anecdotally that clients abandon assistive devices when they are discharged because they find other ways of doing things that are more personally satisfying.

RESEARCH NOTE

For a closer look at how therapists document outcome measures, read how Dale and colleagues (2002) followed five hand therapists who used occupational adaptation to guide therapy. Jack and Estes (2010) provided additional evidence of the efficacy of an occupational adaptation approach in upper extremity practice, and Bachman (2016) described using an occupational adaptation perspective for treating lateral epicondylitis. This is one example of a progression of evidence that contributes to the knowledge base of applying occupational adaptation to upper extremity rehabilitation. Go to https://twu.edu/oaal/ to see an annotated bibliography describing the growing body of research that applies occupational adaptation to children in pediatric practice, adults following a stroke, individuals with mental health concerns, and more.

STORY 6-1

The Gymnast

My personal experience related to relative mastery occurred while I was a collegiate gymnast at Texas Woman's University. I was fortunate to not only make the team but also to be chosen to compete in my specialty events of the vault and uneven bars throughout the competitive season. As I strived to perform at my personal best in each competition, I realized that my desire to be the last vaulter in the lineup was not being met. Typically, the last position in a team event rotation receives the highest score, hence my motivation to claim that position. My self-evaluation affirmed that I was efficient and effective with my performance of the vaulting skill, and the scores I received from the judges were consistently the same over each competition but not the highest on the team. Throughout the season, I continued to make adaptive responses based on my coaching staff's guidance and teaching to improve my skills and difficulty ratings.

Even though my self-satisfaction was low, the coach's satisfaction was high. My coach was extremely pleased that I was the first vaulter and consistently hit my skill in each competition. Knowing that I could obtain a higher score at the end of our team's lineup was frustrating. I truly desired to receive one of the highest scores on the team. I met with my coach to discuss a different place in the lineup. His response was to keep the lineup the same. My coach continued to explain his rationale; I was setting the bar by insisting the judges give a higher-than-average score to the first competitor. Therefore, if my teammates through the lineup continued to hit their vault skills, the scores would build, providing our team with a high event team score. My consistency was keeping the team's score high.

Understanding my contribution and impact on the team's success offered me a different perspective. In past experiences, my mastery of gymnastics events was based on personal scores compared to other competitors; high scores equated to mastery. For example, when my vault score was the highest in the competition, I received first place overall. However, the individual mastery I desired conflicted with the needs of the team, and this realization helped me shift to a high sense of relative mastery in my role as a team member. This press for mastery as an individual gymnast had been met, and the new challenge was to perform as a team member rather than as a sole competitor.

This life experience has altered the way I approach my management duties today. I have experienced this relative mastery throughout my career as an occupational therapist and small business owner because of the internal adaptation process. My continued belief that we are stronger as a team rather than as individuals has guided my therapy practice, clinical skills, and administrative role throughout my career.

Story contributed by Sarah Rupp-Blanchard, OTD, MHA, OTR

One important thing to remember from a therapeutic standpoint is that you are attempting to intervene in the client's internal adaptation process. Allowing the client to assess their progress in terms of the experience of relative mastery provides them with a tool for evaluating occupational responses after the therapy is over and they return home. The case of The Breadwinner (Case 6-1) illustrates how an experience of relative mastery in a routine task generalized to improved performance in a highly valued occupational role.

Because relative mastery is idiosyncratic to the individual, the individual determines what constitutes the extent to which they have experienced efficiency, effectiveness, and satisfaction to self and others. The individual considers the occupational role demands (internal and external) for the activity in question and reaches a personal conclusion about their experience of relative mastery. As an overall assessment of the occupational event (the plan for the response, the response itself, and the outcome), the individual is thought to place the event somewhere on a conceptual continuum between occupational adaptation and occupational dysadaptation with homeostasis as a midpoint. In other words, from awareness of the challenge to the formation of an action plan and experience of the outcome, the individual concludes that their interaction with the occupational environment was somewhere between a "disaster" and a "triumph." The information gained from this self-assessment indicates to the client whether further adaptation is needed. Sometimes this process is drawn out over time, and sometimes it occurs in the blink of an eye.

For an example of how the client's assessment of relative mastery can be used therapeutically, see the case of The Florist (Case 6-2). The Florist illustrates how the client's assessment of relative mastery led to self-directed changes in his intervention plan.

CASE 6-1

The Breadwinner

José was a 56-year-old man who had a left hemisphere stroke 2 months before our encounter. After hospitalization and inpatient rehabilitation, José began attending an outpatient neurorehabilitation center daily. José was the main breadwinner in his home where he lived with his wife and two middle school–aged children. He worked for a large tortilla company delivering tortillas to area grocery stores and arranging the tortilla displays. José had immigrated to the United States from Mexico 10 years ago and spoke Spanish. José's primary concern was the prospect of losing his job and the ability to provide for his family.

José was right-hand dominant and was primarily affected by his stroke in his right upper extremity. He was able to walk independently. His speech was affected minimally, but he was very quiet, and he had little interaction with the other clients because of the language barrier. José displayed a flat affect and engaged in therapeutic exercises but was hesitant to engage in groups or any functional activities. He stated he just wanted his hand to be back to normal and that he wanted to get better but saw no point in games or cooking activities. He would use his affected right arm for theraputty or lifting weights but typically cradled his arm in front of him and avoided using it for any functional activity unless directed to do so.

In a session during the third week at the therapy center, a group of patients were working in the community garden on a hot day. José was primarily using his left hand to water some plants silently, and he was not engaged with the others who were looking for produce to harvest. On the way inside, he slowed by the drink machine and turned toward it as if to get himself a quick drink. He stopped and then turned away to head back to the gym. The therapist noticed his interest and inquired if he was thirsty. He admitted he was thirsty, but he wanted to wait until he could use his straw cup near his desk area. The therapist encouraged him to try getting a drink here because there was a variety of soft drinks from which to choose. He looked at the therapist sideways and sighed dejectedly, knowing this was part of his therapy. He knew the therapist was watching, so he hesitantly used his right hand to grasp a Styrofoam cup and filled the cup partially with soda from the drink machine. He very slowly and carefully brought the cup to his mouth and drank, only using his left hand to assist when his right hand began tremoring halfway through quenching his thirst. His face broke out into a large grin; he had thought he would not be able to drink from the cup, but he had been successful.

The next day at therapy, José came to report to the therapist that during his work shift that morning, he had been practicing picking up each bag of tortillas with his right hand and placing it carefully on the shelf. From then on, with each functional activity, he was much more engaged and asked questions about how participating in the activity might impact his abilities in his work role of arranging tortillas.

ANALYSIS

José's desire for mastery was sparked as he passed the drink machine and realized he was thirsty. The environment presented a demand for mastery with the physical context presenting Styrofoam cups placed at tabletop level next to the drink machine, which was conveniently placed along the path we were walking. The temporal context also came into play; we walked right past this drink machine after a hot gardening activity when José was thirsty. Together, these contextual factors created a press for mastery, calling for an occupational response from José; the occupational challenge was for him to get himself a drink. The context played a large part in initiating this successful interaction for José. He had many opportunities to engage in functional activities throughout his time at the program, but something about the total context of this activity created a press for mastery that sparked an action in him to try this activity as he responded to his role of being able to meet his own basic needs. As he evaluated his adaptive response to this occupational challenge, he had a successful feeling of relative mastery. He was more efficient than he had originally guessed he might be, was able to effectively obtain a drink of soda using his right hand, and was satisfied with the successful completion of this event. His evaluation of efficiency, effectiveness, and satisfaction were all components of his sense of relative mastery. As a result of the activation of José's occupational adaptation process and his experience of increased relative mastery, José generalized the use of his right hand for use during his job for moving tortillas, which was an important occupation for him.

Case and analysis contributed by Anne Sullivan, PhD, OTR

CASE 6-2

The Florist

Mr. Green was a 54-year-old engineer who sustained a bilateral cerebrovascular accident. When first seen by the therapist, he was comatose and unable to engage actively in his intervention. Working closely with Mrs. Green, the therapist learned that Mr. Green enjoyed music and that the Greens owned a flower shop where Mr. Green worked, in addition to his job as an engineer. In the early stages, intervention consisted of occupational readiness activities on the part of the therapist and Mrs. Green. The plan consisted of bilateral upper and lower extremity passive range of motion exercises, sitting balance activities, and sensory stimulation. Mr. Green proved to be responsive to vestibular stimulation, slow rocking, icing, and auditory stimulation, such as bells and the therapist singing songs by a popular singer who was known to be liked by Mr. Green. Mrs. Green was given instructions in passive range of motion, and positioning techniques were taught to nursing staff and Mr. Green's family. By week 3, following surgery and medication, Mr. Green made excellent progress and was able to actively engage in his program. Mr. Green indicated tearfully that he wanted to make a special flower arrangement for his wife to celebrate their upcoming anniversary. Thus, his occupational role as a florist became the guide to intervention, and the therapist was able to emphasize occupational activity that was relevant to the role of the florist.

The therapist educated herself by conducting an activity analysis of flower arranging and obtained a supply of silk flowers. She consulted with Mrs. Green as well for insight into how she and Mr. Green carried out the activities of flower arranging in their business.

Mr. Green began planning and making weekly floral arrangements while he was responding and adapting to the changes in his person system brought on by the cerebrovascular accident. Each week Mr. Green evaluated his progress in relative mastery (efficiency, effectiveness, and satisfaction to self/others). As a result of these weekly self-evaluations, Mr. Green made the following adjustments to his intervention plan:

- For more efficiency, during the session before the one in which he was to create a flower arrangement, he planned first in his mind and then on paper the particular arrangement he wanted to create.
- He began taking weekly pictures to see his improvements, which resulted in greater satisfaction to himself.
- Mrs. Green began leaving the arrangements he had made at the nurses' station for the weekend to reinforce feelings of satisfaction to society.
- He requested a more rigorous room exercise program to increase his endurance and strength.
- He borrowed flower books to re-educate himself for an increased feeling of effectiveness.
- Before transfer to a rehabilitation setting, Mr. Green began to help one of the nurses plan the flowers for her wedding.

Case contributed by Melissa McClung, MOT, OTR

The goal of including the client in self-evaluation of their progress is two-fold. First, it can assist them in identifying improvement and their contribution to that improved status. Second, the capacity to evaluate their responses when therapy ends is an empowerment tool that can assist them in all areas of occupational life to identify when their responses are satisfactory and when they need to be changed. The lack of an ability to evaluate one's responses can result in perseveration of dysadaptive behavior with extended and sometimes very dysfunctional outcomes.

Dysadaptation is not always due to a lack of self-evaluation; sometimes it is a product of faulty self-evaluation. If relative mastery does not align with mastery when issues of safety are involved, reality testing needs to come into play. Reality testing can happen when the therapist skillfully acts as an agent of the environment to help the client discover a faulty sense of relative mastery that may put them in danger (e.g., using a simulated or modified task so that mistakes are not perilous [a driving simulator, a plastic knife to cut a banana, a large blunt needle for sewing through precut holes, and so on]). In the case of cognitive impairment or delay that prevents insight or heightened awareness, we further modify the environment or task to maintain safety.

Be aware that a single success is not necessarily an indication that a person's occupational adaptation process is fully functioning and no longer requires attention or intervention. Elaina DaLomba (occupational therapist and occupational adaptation scholar) shared that, in her practice with school children, she "always wanted to see the behavior, or the action that we want, in many different environments, not just in that one classroom where I pushed in. You know, [I look for carry-over] in PE [physical education] and in the lunchroom

… " She continued by cautioning, "You know it's not mastery if you can only do it when you have all the scaffolding around you" (L. Figueroa, personal communication, March 13, 2019). Recall that in the guiding principles for intervention (see Table 1-1), indicators that an adaptive response has been integrated include (a) spontaneous generalization to other activities, (b) initiation of new approaches in novel situations, and (c) an increase in relative mastery.

Keep in mind that a shift from a novel challenge in primary energy with low relative mastery to secondary energy with high relative mastery can happen very rapidly; let us use knot tying as an example. I (CLE) watched a YouTube video of how to tie a specific knot (demand) that I recently wanted (desire) to use on a project (press from an occupational challenge). I watched the 18-second demo over and over (about six times), tried to tie the knot two or three times but failed

(low relative mastery), went back to the video to see where I went wrong (strong desire), and then tried again with eventual success—all on primary energy with a high degree of relative mastery. After my first successful attempt, I experienced an immediate rise in my sense of relative mastery and repeated the knot several times (still on primary energy) to make sure I would not forget it. Within 3 to 5 minutes, I could tie the knot while having a conversation or watching TV (secondary energy) with a high degree of relative mastery. However, sometimes gaining relative mastery takes persistence and assistance over time, as in the case of The Student Intern (Case 6-3).

An intern has a strong desire for mastery that will lead to degree completion and a professional career. The demands for mastery are also high; the academic institution must ensure that interns meet accreditation standards and eligibility

---

CASE 6-3

The Student Intern

While working at an equine-assisted therapy program, I was a clinical instructor to a Level II fieldwork student in her first rotation. She had been working on improving communication during therapy sessions. Because of the dynamic nature of coordinating multiple components of hippotherapy, the therapist is responsible for communicating with the client, side walkers, and horse handlers. Poor communication with any of these individuals may result in unproductive treatment sessions.

When Annie first started her rotation, she was very shy, timid, and self-conscious about her abilities. During the first few weeks, the treatment sessions required that she practice leading; without a lead nobody would do anything, including the horse. She was very eager to do her best and slowly began taking over calling commands to the side walker and horse handler. After treatment sessions, she would express discontent because of the multitasking demands and not feeling effective or that she was being efficient with her time. She would often focus primarily on the patient and forget to call commands or vice versa, which affected therapeutic interventions.

At the end of every week, Annie was asked to reflect on her perceived strengths, weaknesses, and areas for improvement. Those areas for improvement along with newly targeted objectives then became the focus for the following week.

Until week 4, she had to focus and concentrate when attempting to orchestrate all the moving parts during treatment sessions, experiencing only low levels of relative mastery, but by week 8, Annie was able to effortlessly call commands to the horse handlers and prompt side walkers while attending to the needs of the rider. By the time she was nearing the end of her rotation, she demonstrated the ability to process feedback and modify her responses using techniques that worked previously, as well as new techniques based on feedback. She had shifted concentration and focus during sessions to the hands-on aspects of targeted interventions to support client goals.

As a result of her progress, Annie was more efficient with her time and resources. Her efficiency allowed her clients to be more engaged during sessions because she required less focus on calling commands. She also expressed satisfaction with her performance as she recognized that she was developing her clinical reasoning skills, confidence, and achieving targeted objectives set for the week. Her occupational response to her role expectations allowed her to expand her skills, and in turn, create adaptive responses that she could then incorporate into her adaptation repertoire.

Case contributed by Alondra Ammon, MOT, OTR/L

NEURO SPOTLIGHT

Resilience

Resilience is a specific aspect of the adaptive response evaluation process that manifests as physiological and behavioral adaptation to internal or external stressors. From a physiological perspective, resilience refers to mechanisms that support survival and well-being through homeostasis. Resilience is the ability of the central nervous system and the body to minimize allostatic load and successfully adapt to stressors.

There is a growing body of research on the neurochemical mechanisms of stress that shows several processes and neurochemicals involved in the mediation of stress, including serotonin receptors, neuropeptide Y, and the hypothalamic-pituitary-adrenal (HPA) axis. The HPA axis is a series of connections that mediate the effects of stress on the central nervous system, the physiological processes of the body, and the resulting behavior related to stress. The HPA axis produces hormonal, neurochemical, and physiological alterations that are spread throughout, and therefore, are influential across brain and body structures and functions. Using the HPA axis, glucocorticoids are released from the adrenal glands and transmitted to higher-level structures, such as the hippocampus, amygdala, medial prefrontal cortex, and other limbic and midbrain structures. These structures, through glucosteroid expression, generate or regulate the behavioral responses that are seen in response to stress.

Long-term or chronic stress maintains activation of the HPA axis. Over time, this continued activation of the HPA axis has an effect on the body that contributes myriad behavioral and physical health issues, including anxiety, depressive disorders, post-traumatic stress disorder, increased hypertension, immunosuppression, osteoporosis, insulin resistance, obesity, and cardiovascular disease.

Lastly, in the adaptive response processes, individuals with different psychiatric conditions will respond and adapt in various ways. The adaptive responses in people with behavioral health conditions is partially linked to changes in desire for mastery or motivation and may be related to deficits in motivation. Considering two distinct behavioral health conditions, schizophrenia and depression, there are differences in the adaptive response patterns that are generated by differences in neurologic processes. People with depression have impairments in capacity for anticipation, learning, effort, and happiness (hedonia). In contrast, patients with schizophrenia have difficulty translating reward experience to anticipation and action selection. Each of these adaptive response patterns is directly linked to the central nervous system structures and processes that underlie each condition.

RECOMMENDED READINGS

Barch, D. M. (2005). The cognitive neuroscience of schizophrenia. *Annual Review of Clinical Psychology, 1,* 321-353. https://doi.org/10.1146/annurev.clinpsy.1.102803.143959

Davidson, R. J., Pizzagalli, D., Nitschke, J. B., & Putnam, K. (2002). Depression: Perspectives from affective neuroscience. *Annual Review of Psychology, 53*(1), 545-574. https://doi.org/10.1146/annurev.psych.53.100901.135148

Guidi, J., Lucente, M., Sonino, N., & Fava, G. A. (2021). Allostatic load and its impact on health: A systematic review. *Psychotherapy and Psychosomatics, 90,* 11-27. https://doi.org/10.1159/000510696

Maniam, J., Antoniadis, C., & Morris, M. J. (2014). Early-life stress, HPA axis adaptation, and mechanisms contributing to later health outcomes. *Frontiers in Endocrinology, 5,* 73. https://doi.org/10.3389/fendo.2014.00073

Romero, M. L., & Butler, L. K. (2007). Endocrinology of stress. *International Journal of Comparative Psychology, 20*(2), 89-95.

requirements for credentialing and licensure, and the fieldwork site has expectations that their clients will receive a high standard of care. The press for mastery comes in the form of daily challenges to produce adaptive responses while caring for the individual needs of clients, each within their unique circumstances and contexts. Relative mastery can be experienced in individual tasks and with clients numerous times throughout the days and weeks, and ultimately, the intern hopes to complete the rotation with a high sense of relative mastery within the role of the occupational therapist in a particular setting.

A Deeper Dive

In his 1999 Eleanor Clarke Slagle lecture, Dr. Charles Christiansen presented his ideas on occupation as identity. He made three summary statements about symbolic interactionism that relate well to occupational adaptation:

(a) We communicate symbolically much of the time and that the language of social life consists of both spoken and unspoken messages; (b) through our conversations with ourselves, we are able to modify our behaviors to gain social approval; and (c) the need for social approval encourages conformity, which promotes stability and predictability, but occasionally also yields individual creativity that, when adopted, serves to advance the social group. (Christiansen, 1999, p. 551)

When we accept an occupational challenge, we communicate our desire for mastery and acknowledge both internal and external expectations. In occupational adaptation terms, we modify our adaptive response behaviors to reach a level of efficiency and effectiveness that satisfies both self and others. We agree and affirm that satisfaction to others is gauged against external expectations and that we tend to seek homeostasis by repeating successful adaptive strategies. However, novelty and shifting contexts often create a press for mastery that requires a modified or new (creative) adaptive response. When witnessed by others, adaptive responses add to a collective adaptation gestalt that serves to raise a group's relative mastery as well (McKay et al., 2021).

TAKE-AWAY MESSAGES

◊ Relative mastery is an internal self-evaluation of efficiency, effectiveness, and satisfaction to self and others.

◊ The therapist can facilitate a conscious self-evaluation of relative mastery to enable the occupational adaptation process.

◊ An increasing sense of relative mastery is a source of motivation that fuels the desire for mastery and raises internal expectations for success with occupational challenges.

References

Bachman, S. (2016). Evidence-based approach to treating lateral epicondylitis using the occupational adaptation model. *American Journal of Occupational Therapy, 70*(2), 7002360010. https://doi.org/10.5014/ajot.2016.016972

Christiansen, C. H. (1999). Defining lives: Occupation as identity: An essay on competence, coherence, and the creation of meaning, 1999 Eleanor Clarke Slagle lecture. *American Journal of Occupational Therapy, 53*(6), 547-558. https://doi.org/10.5014/ajot.53.6.547

Dale, L. M., Fabrizio, A. J., Adhlakha, P., Mahon, M. K., McGraw, E. E., Neyenhaus, R. D., Sledd, T., & Zaber, J. M. (2002). Occupational therapists working in hand therapy: The practice of holism in a cost containment environment. *Work, 19*(1), 35-45.

Jack, J., & Estes, R. I. (2010). Documenting progress: Hand therapy treatment shift from biomechanical to occupational adaptation. *American Journal of Occupational Therapy, 64*(1), 82-87. https://doi.org/10.5014/ajot.64.1.82

McKay, M. H., Pickens, N., Medley, A., Cooper, D. H., & Evetts, C. (2021). Comparing occupational adaptation-based and traditional training programs for dementia care teams: An embedded mixed-methods study. *Gerontologist, 61*(4), 582-594. https://doi.org/10.1093/geront/gnaa160

Try It On

Until now, you have been focusing on the generation or creation of your response. Reflect on the response you actually executed. Now it's time for you to evaluate that response. Relative mastery, a hallmark of occupational adaptation, relates to your perception of how efficient, effective, and satisfying to self and society your response was. Think about your challenge once again and evaluate your sense of relative mastery.

	CIRCLE ONE OF THE FOLLOWING IN EACH CATEGORY				
RELATIVE MASTERY	**1 (LOW)**	**2**	**3**	**4**	**5 (HIGH)**
Efficiency How well did you use your time, energy, and resources while you were engaging in responding to your challenge?	1	2	3	4	5
Effectiveness To what extent did you accomplish what you set out to do?	1	2	3	4	5
Satisfaction to self and others How much satisfaction did you experience with your response?	1	2	3	4	5
How about others?	1	2	3	4	5

So now you've been faced with an occupational challenge. You've generated a plan to meet the challenge and responded. You have evaluated your response. Lastly, you need to focus on how you integrate this occupational event into your overall capacity for adaptation. Chapter 7 deals with this integration action.

CHAPTER 7

Adaptive Response Integration, Adaptive Repertoire

How Has the Person Changed or Adapted?

> *Adaptation is an inherently cumulative process in which the past shapes the future ... The concept of adaptation thus prompts therapists to think not only about change, but also about continuity in the lives of our clients.*
> —Jean Cole Spencer and colleagues (1996, p. 527)

Following the adaptive response evaluation, synthesis of the occupational event and its integration into the person system becomes the work of the adaptive response integration subprocess. It is in the action of this integration that the adaptation process culminates. This is the point at which the occupational challenge and its subsequent response impacts the individual's state of occupational functioning. In other words, this is when all the information in the occupational event becomes translated and stored in a form that the person can use in the future. We call this accumulation of adaptation experiences an *adaptive repertoire*.

The concept of an adaptive repertoire focuses on client strengths (Spencer et al., 1996). When encountering significant occupational challenges, remembering that we have responded adaptively in the past can fuel our hopes for the future, boosting internal expectations for success and increasing our desire for mastery. Examination of one's adaptive repertoire can also reveal gaps or limitations in performance skills or patterns. Under another theoretical frame of reference, a therapist might see this as a need for skill building through teaching and exercise. By contrast, in occupational adaptation, we propose that adaptation is more likely to be integrated into a repertoire that will enable generalized success beyond the current circumstance when we tap into the client's desire for mastery and orchestrate a just-right challenge that reinforces the adaptation process.

Evetts, C. L., & Baxter, M. F. *Cases and Concepts in Occupational Adaptation: Translating Theory into Action* (pp. 67-72).
DOI: 10.4324/9781003522850-7

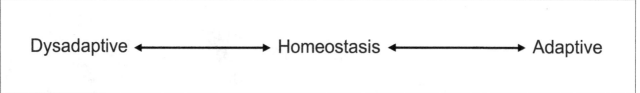

Figure 7-1. Adaptation continuum.

Occupational adaptation suggests that one of three states of occupational functioning will be strengthened or reinforced in the person because of adaptive response integration: occupational adaptation, homeostasis, or occupational dysadaptation. An adaptation response exists on a continuum between adaptive and dysadaptive with homeostasis in the middle (Figure 7-1).

You are probably more accustomed to hearing the term *maladaptive*, which is defined as relating to incomplete, inadequate, or faulty adaptation. The prefix "mal" means "bad, wrongful, or ill." When we look at the adaptive continuum, we see the far side of adaptation as dysadaptation. Dysadaptation refers to the inability to satisfactorily accommodate in response to change. Therefore, with homeostasis representing stability (no change), a skillful response to an occupational challenge is deemed adaptive (a response that is more toward positive change with a higher sense of relative mastery). On the other side of the continuum, a response that is unsatisfactory, inadequate, or leads to potential harm is considered less adaptive or dysadaptive.

The memory of an occupational event activates the integration process to store the response in the person's adaptive repertoire. This memory is an essential precursor to what change, if any, develops. In other words, if the individual is to respond to similar challenges in the future, what might that individual do differently to respond more masterfully? What did the individual learn about the relationship between how the occupational response was created and the outcome it produced? If the individual's assessment of their response was that it did produce a positive experience of relative mastery, then the state of occupational adaptation will be strengthened. Perhaps only minor adjustments in planning similar responses in the future will produce even better results. Perhaps no change is needed. If, because of their assessment, the individual found that the experience of relative mastery was more negative than positive, major adjustments may be necessary for the future to produce satisfactory results. If the individual recognizes the dysadaptive nature of the response and still produces no change in the way similar subsequent challenges are confronted, then the state of occupational dysadaptation will be reinforced.

Can a dysadaptive response ever lead to a strengthening of the state of occupational adaptation? Indeed, it can. Aversive events can be very powerful stimuli for adaptation.

When the person, through the action of adaptive response evaluation, concludes that they do not want to experience low relative mastery in the future, significant change can occur. A simple example might be a student who neglects to study for a test and then receives a failing grade on it. Although poor study habits may reflect dysadaptive behavior, when the adaptation process is functioning at its best, reflecting on the experience could encourage better practices before the next examination. Thus, the unpleasant experience leads to adaptation. However, people whose occupational adaptation process is dysfunctional may be unable to take advantage of the push for adaptation present in adverse events. It may be necessary for them to continue responding in dysadaptive ways (e.g., with existing hyperstable responses) until adaptive response evaluation and integration subprocesses can function more successfully. The individual who does not engage in the evaluation and integration functions will continue to respond in dysfunctional ways because the necessary functions of these important subprocesses are not operating effectively, or in some cases, not operating at all.

Let us return for a moment to Jill, our new mother in Chapter 1 (Story 1-1). Her initial experience of low levels of relative mastery did not lead to change even though adaptation was needed. She decided to repeat the same dysfunctional actions. She would simply "try harder." She may have to cycle through the process several times before reaching an awareness that substantial change is in order. If her occupational adaptation process is functioning well, she will likely be able to make adaptations that will enhance her experience of relative mastery. A hopeful sign is that she did evaluate her response. Her capacity to evaluate appears intact.

When the adaptive response integration subprocess is functioning well, adaptation is most likely to occur. If the goal of intervention is to address an individual's internal adaptation process, what are the indicators that this internal process has actually been impacted? The following are indicators that the occupational adaptation process is functioning as the individual confronts and responds to occupational challenges:

- The client experiences increased relative mastery as they respond to occupational challenges.
- The client demonstrates spontaneous generalizations to novel tasks without prompting by the therapist or others.
- The client initiates adaptations not previously seen or specifically suggested.

NEURO SPOTLIGHT

Stress

There is a growing body of research on the neurochemical mechanisms of stress that shows several processes and neurochemicals involved in the mediation of stress, including serotonin receptors, neuropeptide Y, and the hypothalamic-pituitary-adrenal (HPA) axis. The HPA axis is a series of connections that mediate the effects of stress on the central nervous system, the physiological processes of the body, and the resulting behavior related to stress. The HPA axis produces hormonal, neurochemical, and physiological alterations that are spread throughout, and therefore, are influential across brain and body structures and functions. Long-term stress and impairments with an imbalance of serotonin, neuropeptide Y, and the effects related to HPA activation impart substantial demands for adaptation on the neural systems and the body. Long-term stress and impaired ability to adapt lead to myriad behavioral and physical health issues, including anxiety, depressive disorders, post-traumatic stress disorder, increased hypertension, immunosuppression, osteoporosis, insulin resistance, obesity, and cardiovascular disease.

RECOMMENDED READINGS

Karin, O., Raz, M., Tendler, A., Bar, A., Kohanim, Y. K., Milo, T., Alon, U. (2020). A new model for the HPA axis explains dysregulation of stress hormones on the timescale of weeks. *Molecular Systems Biology, 16,* e9510. https://doi.org/10.15252/msb.20209510

Young, E. S., Doom, J. R., Farrell, A. K., Carlson, E. A., Englund, M. M., Miller, G. E., Gunnar, M. R., Roisman, G. I., & Simpson, J. A. (2021). Life stress and cortisol reactivity: An exploratory analysis of the effects of stress exposure across life on HPA-axis functioning. *Development and Psychopathology, 33*(1), 301-312. https://doi.org/10.1017/S0954579419001779

All three of these indicators point to internal factors at work. The case of The Special Forces Veteran (Case 7-1) illustrates how the concept of a strong adaptation repertoire can explain unexpected, enhanced recovery after serious trauma.

The case of The Older Homemaker (Case 7-2) illustrates spontaneous generalization and initiation of adaptation. This client exemplifies indicators of the internal adaptation process at work. The client experienced increasing relative mastery throughout therapy. As she did so, she upgraded her goals. She also demonstrated spontaneous generalization of skills to tasks and self-initiated adaptations. This case illustrates how the client can direct the course of therapy with the help of a therapist when intervention is focused on occupational activities that are meaningful to the individual.

Recall that anticipating potential outcomes, both good and bad, promotes more adaptive and masterful responses. Some scholars have argued that high levels of cognitive processing are required to anticipate the consequences of one's actions, especially in novel situations. Therefore, the following question emerges: Is the adaptive response process inherently limited for individuals with cognitive deficits? Theoretically speaking, the concept of an adaptive repertoire that is available as a person generates an adaptive response through their adaptation gestalt solves this dilemma. If we can build a robust adaptive repertoire by providing a rich array of opportunities (occupational challenges) to generate, evaluate, and integrate adaptive responses that lead to relative mastery, then the internal adaptation process is strengthened. The person can call on resources beyond cognition (i.e., muscle memory and habit training) to respond adaptively despite less-than-robust cognitive processing.

A Deeper Dive

For an extended case study of a person with severe brain injury, read Dr. Gordon Giles's 2018 Eleanor Clarke Slagle lecture. Dr. Giles weaves a story throughout this lecture, and your challenge is to apply principles of occupational adaptation to Dave. The following is a teaser:

> We had deliberately taught Dave two specific skills, personal hygiene and how to make breakfast, but we soon learned that we had accidentally taught him a generic strategy—when you don't know what to do, look for instructions—because when he became confused in a situation, that is exactly what he did; he looked for instructions. So we started to leave written instructions all over the place so that when he became confused, he would find the instructions and then follow them. (Giles, 2018, p. 8)

Remember "occupational adaptation is a way to name and frame what good therapists do" (J. Schkade, personal communication, April 30, 1993). Therefore, when you hear about really good occupation-based therapy, it is not hard to apply the concepts within occupational adaptation theory to explain what happened in the internal adaptation process.

CASE 7-1

The Special Forces Veteran

As a rehabilitation specialist at a Veterans Affairs hospital, I accepted a consult from the physical medicine and rehabilitation department for a name I recognized. I had treated the veteran 2 years prior for a ruptured distal bicep tendon. When I say "treated," I mean I gave him a protocol and some therapy bands and sent him on his way because he had a job he had been called out on and needed to leave the next day. I held my breath as I watched him go, although I knew in the back of my mind I did not need to hold my breath too long because he was special forces, and my experience with those guys is that they were a little like Wolverine from X-Men (Marvel Comics): able to put up with a lot and heal fast.

However, when I read the history on the new consult, my heart sank—polytrauma. He had been in an accident that resulted in him being placed in a medically induced coma for 3 months, extensive surgeries to repair internal organs, neurologic damage to his right upper extremity, traumatic brain injury, and a shattered right hip. When he arrived for his initial occupational therapy evaluation, I did not recognize him. The literal giant of a man I had sent on his way to who knows where with a couple of therapy bands arrived back to the clinic at least 125 pounds lighter and being pushed in a wheelchair.

During the evaluation, I learned that he had checked himself out of the inpatient rehabilitation unit he was in because he did not get the rehabilitative care he believed he needed. He stated that he did not want to be treated in a civilian facility either, that he needed to be with other service members and people who understood who he was and where he came from. After performing the objective assessment during which I found limitations in all areas of activities of daily living because of right upper extremity spasticity, mild cognitive deficits (most to attention and short-term memory), and limitations to all transfers due to right lower extremity spasticity and healing hip fracture, we talked about his goals. He stated that he wished to walk his daughter down the aisle in 1 month and return to full duty. I gulped, knowing the chances were slight that he would meet either of those goals. Looking back, I should not have doubted that it was an option or a probability. As it turns out, he was out of the garage-sale special wheelchair he had bought on his own and using a walker by the time the specialized wheelchair we had ordered for him arrived 1 week later. Within 1 month, he did walk his daughter down the aisle with the use of a cane. When I reassessed his cognition at the 8-week follow-up, he was functioning within normal limits. He was discharged to a home program after 12 weeks of therapy.

Just about 3 months later, he showed up again in my clinic to say hi, to thank me, and to let me know that he had been approved to return to full duty where he was functioning just fine. I told him there were no thanks needed because he had done the work himself, and I meant it. Seeing this veteran again made me wonder why it is that my special forces guys do so much better in therapy than my other clients.

As a general rule, I can expect a quicker adaptive response in my clients who come from special forces communities. This can be explained by an integrated adaptive response mechanism that responds quickly and dynamically to changes in environmental demands. I believe that these clients have personal factors and client factors that predispose them to be able to withstand highly stressful environmental contexts. At the same time, the fact that they completed training and have operated in combat situations leads me to believe their adaptive responses in those situations have further integrated positive occupational adaptation responses (into a robust adaptive repertoire) that have helped them to respond adaptively to many different occupational challenges.

Case contributed by Christine E. Haines, PhD, OTR

FUTURE RESEARCH

The Special Forces Veteran is a case of an extremely adaptive individual. Was he adaptive because of his training, or did he survive and excel in the training because he was so adaptive? We would first need to dig deep into the existing research (e.g., on resilience) to formulate appropriate research questions in answering this which-came-first inquiry.

CASE 7-2 ──

The Older Homemaker

Mrs. Johnson was a 66-year-old woman with uncontrolled diabetes. She had been found unconscious and subsequently hospitalized. Before this time, she had become progressively bedbound and had not walked for 3 months before the hospitalization. In addition to being severely malnourished and debilitated (she weighed less than 80 pounds), she had been consuming a bottle of bourbon every 2 days for some time. She was diagnosed with diabetic ketoacidosis and peripheral neuropathy. She lived alone with her adult son, who was infrequently employed and sometimes undependable. Upon discharge from the hospital, she was referred to a home health agency for occupational therapy.

During the first occupational therapy session, an interview was conducted, and goals were set. At the next visit, Mrs. Johnson sat at the side of the bed briefly while the therapist explored her interests. Mrs. Johnson indicated that she had been a talented craftswoman but no longer cared to engage in that activity because of failing eyesight and loss of sensation in her fingertips because of peripheral neuropathy. She did agree that at the next session she would sit in a wheelchair and play cards. When, in session three, it was time to transfer to the wheelchair, Mrs. Johnson was apprehensive about the therapist's ability to safely carry out the transfer. The therapist explained the mechanics of the transfer, including the concept of weight shifting. Mrs. Johnson was able to transfer with minimal assistance and was pleased with how smoothly the transfer was accomplished. She sat in the chair for 1 hour playing cards and expressed pleasure with this accomplishment (increased relative mastery).

In session four, Mrs. Johnson transferred with minimal assistance. At her request, the client and therapist moved to the kitchen, which was piled high with dirty dishes and trash. Together, they put dishes in the dishwasher and cleaned countertops. Mrs. Johnson volunteered that if her coffee can and filters were placed lower, she could make coffee by herself (self-initiated adaptation). In session five, the therapist suggested that they work on transferring from the bed to the bedside commode. Mrs. Johnson informed the therapist that she had already been doing that by herself (spontaneous generalization). She also informed the physical therapist that she had stood at the kitchen sink for 3 minutes during occupational therapy. As a result, the physical therapist ordered a walker, and gait training progressed rapidly.

In subsequent sessions, Mrs. Johnson baked corn bread, made soup, and asked to sweep the kitchen floor. Her next goal was to transfer to the bottom of her bathtub. The therapist reported that throughout intervention there were many updated goals as Mrs. Johnson's confidence grew and her goals became more ambitious. Thus, Mrs. Johnson was directing the course of therapy as a result of her internal occupational adaptation process at work. She was evaluating the outcome of her occupational response and selecting the next occupational challenge.

Case based on Ford (1995)

TAKE-AWAY MESSAGES

◊ If we intervene too quickly by solving problems for our clients, we may rob them of an opportunity to experience themselves as masterful agents of change. It is empowering to be able to say, "I did it myself."

◊ Both successful and less-than-satisfying responses to occupational challenges can contribute to an adaptation repertoire that fuels future success.

◊ We can observe the adaptation process at work as a client experiences increased relative mastery, demonstrates spontaneous generalizations, and initiates novel adaptations.

References

Ford, K. (1995). Occupational adaptation in home health: A therapist's viewpoint. *Home Health & Community Special Interest Section Newsletter, 2*(1), 2-4.

Giles, G. M. (2018). 2018 Eleanor Clarke Slagle lecture—Neurocognitive rehabilitation: Skills or strategies? *American Journal of Occupational Therapy, 72,* 7206150010. https://doi.org/10.5014/ajot.2018.726001

Spencer, J. C., Davidson, H. A., & White, V. K. (1996). Continuity and change: Past experience as adaptive repertoire in occupational adaptation. *American Journal of Occupational Therapy, 50*(7), 526-534. https://doi.org/10.5014/ajot.50.7.526

Try It On

You've been busy in this section of the book. You've generated a response for your challenge, responded, and evaluated your response. The following activity will guide you toward identifying factors for integration.

Adaptive Response Integration

Learning

Reflecting on your challenge, think about your expectations. How did your plan compare to your actual response to the challenge?

Now, reflect on your sense of relative mastery (efficiency, effectiveness, and satisfaction to self and others). What did you learn?

Modification of the Person System

When faced with the same challenge, what would you do differently? Would the difference be your expectation (perhaps how you generated or planned your response)?

The occupational adaptation process continues, and the environment is the next focal point.

CHAPTER 8

Assessment by the Occupational Environment, Incorporation into the Occupational Environment

How Does the Environment Respond?

When one tugs at a single thing in nature,
[one] finds it attached to the rest of the world.
—John Muir

The Internal Occupational Adaptation Process

The internal occupational adaptation process is characterized by the individual interacting holistically with the occupational environment through occupational challenges. The person must recognize that a challenge exists and perceive both internal and external role expectations. With these perceptions guiding the process, the individual generates an occupational response. Upon expression of the response, the individual then evaluates its impact in terms of the extent to which relative mastery was experienced. Following evaluation, the individual synthesizes the occupational event, and the results become integrated into the person as learning and adaptation.

Evetts, C. L., & Baxter, M. F. *Cases and Concepts in Occupational Adaptation:*
Translating Theory into Action (pp. 73-79).
DOI: 10.4324/9781003522850-8

Evaluation by the Occupational Environment

The discussion thus far has centered on the individual responding to an occupational challenge. The occupational environment is an active participant during the occupational adaptation process. The occupational environment contributes substantially to the nature of the occupational challenge and, on occasion, may be the primary determinant of the characteristics in which the challenge appears. It has a profound impact on the occupational role expectations because it functions as the source of expectations external to the individual. Through the actions of the physical, social, and cultural aspects of the environment, external expectations take on shape, texture, and tone. Thus, the influence of the environmental context carries great importance for the individual desiring to produce a response to the occupational challenge that is adaptive and masterful. Once an occupational response is produced, the occupational environment also assesses that response and provides feedback relative to the external expectations.

There are indicators of physical, social, and cultural influences involved in the environment's assessment. Because people are part of the social and cultural subsystems, the assessment function is more apparent in those components of the occupational environment. However, parameters of the physical environment may contribute important features that are essential for the individual to note. These physical features can markedly influence the external expectations for an occupational role. Physical attributes convey indications of both possibilities and limitations for the person in preparing and executing an adaptive occupational response. For example, the person engaging in an occupational role requiring the use of certain equipment is both enabled and constrained by the capabilities of that equipment. The cabinet maker operates within the capabilities offered by the available tools. The secretary prepares documents efficiently as enabled by electronic hardware and software with its relative speed and sophistication.

Environmental stimuli, such as the ambient temperature in the workplace, call for the individual to dress for either warm or cold conditions to function optimally. The highway construction worker dresses differently for work under a scorching summer sun and a cold winter wind. The occupational therapist whose daily activity involves assisting clients with physical transfers will wear shoes that provide comfort and stability. The therapist whose function involves the use of leather stains, ceramic glazes, or copper tooling chemicals will recognize artistic possibilities and heed safety protocols in handling caustic substances. The therapist who is responsible for clients on a community outing will want to know features of the terrain, accessibility, and street patterns to lead those clients on a therapeutically successful event. Awareness of the physical features of the occupational environment is critical for the person preparing an occupational response.

The physical environment gives feedback to the individual regarding the satisfactory or unsatisfactory nature of the response. Individuals who fail to note boundaries or hazards present in the physical or nonhuman aspects of the external expectations may place themselves at risk for personal harm at worst and a lack of success in responding to the challenge at best. The feedback is frequently instantaneous, such as a tennis serve placed very precisely within the opponent's court to prevent a return or a cut on the finger from an unexpectedly sharp paring knife.

The social environment gives feedback regarding the extent to which expectations or limitations of the social structure in a particular occupational environment have been met, respected, or violated. When the expectations are clearly delineated, the person's task in meeting those expectations is more easily perceived. In many occupational environments, the social expectations, particularly within informal social structures, may be difficult to identify and plan a satisfactory response. The person who is new to a setting will certainly encounter feedback that indicates how accurately the social system is being perceived and how successfully it is negotiated. Long-standing social networks may be powerful influences and difficult to penetrate for the person wishing to become a part of that social environment. The high school student new to the community and the school may receive clear indications of the extent to which a welcoming atmosphere extends from existing social groups. Early social interactions in the occupational role of student generate feedback regarding success or failure respective to the expectations of the social environment. Likewise, the new employee desiring to be a part of a social environment may find that it is difficult to be included in informal gatherings of that network. This can be particularly true of those gatherings that have become ritualized, such as a group of individuals whose social activities take place over lunch or similar break periods. For a particular occupational environment, awareness of the social system and its properties has the potential to substantially impact one's experience of relative mastery.

The cultural environment can provide some of the most powerful feedback regarding the occupational response. Rules, customs, values, ethical codes, and similar guides provide cues for action and constitute the "rules of the road." These implicit and explicit rules relate to the reason for the environment's existence (i.e., its mission). This is true whether the context be work or school, leisure, or self-care. If education is the mission, as in school settings, there are cultural features that describe the standards and expectations for those engaged in various roles. If the manufacture of a product is the mission, the culture will differ from one workplace to another. For example, a worker engaged in the manufacture of computer chips will encounter a very different culture from a worker engaged in the manufacture of steel. Likewise, in leisure environments, cultures differ. Participation in a softball game involves cultural expectations quite different from those seen in a game of chess. The various components of an occupational environment's culture may come from historical or traditional origins. Some cultural expectations develop as a result of pressures from outside the environment, which impact the ways in which the culture operates (e.g., laws, standards of regulating bodies, or funding sources). Others' expectations emerge from the need for a group of individuals to go about tasks in a systematic or organized manner in order to achieve mission-related goals. Regardless of the makeup of a particular environmental culture, mindful attention to cultural expectations is essential if the individual is to experience positive relative mastery. As with the social environment, there are "keepers" of the culture who will provide feedback to the individual regarding the degree to which the cultural expectations are being met.

The case of The Lineman (Case 8-1) illustrates expectations and input from the occupational environment. As you read, note expectations, input, and feedback on the Case 8-1 Worksheet.

All aspects of the occupational environment, including but not limited to physical, social, and cultural context, evaluate (give feedback regarding) the individual's occupational response. This evaluation feeds back into the occupational environment and becomes incorporated there. The feedback is not compartmentalized, but aspects interact to enrich and bind elements within the greater context. For example, in the case of The Lineman, physical aspects of pee wee football impact the environment in both social and cultural ways. The uniform is a physical object with social impact, and the shape of a football, another physical object, influences cultural expectations (Case 8-1 Worksheet answer key in Appendix B).

CASE 8-1

The Lineman

BACKGROUND

John was a young boy enrolled in second grade of a rural, public elementary school. In the summer after second grade, his mother wished for him to engage in a camp-based experience to develop friendships with similarly aged peers. His mother enrolled him in a 3-week occupational therapy–based camp program. The camp was designed to offer children opportunities to learn specific social skills and strategies to effectively regulate their bodies to support interactions with similarly aged peers.

Before the camp experience, John participated in a 1-hour evaluation with his mother present. During the evaluation, his mother reported that he had a history of behavioral outbursts, such as throwing desks, hitting or pushing others, and screaming. As a result, he had a behavior plan and therapeutic support staff at school who implemented his behavior plan throughout the day. His mother reported that his behaviors had been frequent during kindergarten, and since then, had become fairly well managed. She also did not see these behaviors present in the home environment. John loved to play, read, or watch television about dinosaurs. He wanted to play with others but never had positive experiences. John reportedly dominated conversations with his preferred topics. When he would become frustrated during these interactions, he would either "shut down" or become verbally and, at times, physically aggressive.

John's father supported his desire to play football on a local school team. His mother reported that John often became upset during football practices. He would cry and require reassurance from her on the sideline. In addition, he did not interact with his teammates. John told his mother he wanted to play, but his mother reported concern because she believed this activity produced significant stress for John.

(continued)

John had a desire to develop friendships and be a member of the football team. Although he had a strong desire to fulfill the roles of friend and team member, John's occupational performance was limited by poor self-regulation, decreased motor planning skills, sensitivity to tactile information, and decreased social skills. The environmental demands, specifically a football team's culture, were not in alignment with his current skills. John was expected to practice with his teammates, complete drills, listen to the coaches' directives, engage in team-building exercises, and participate in games. This incongruence between the environmental demands and his skills created an occupational challenge.

John attended a 3-week day camp experience with similarly aged peers. Throughout this camp experience, John became more confident in his interactions with others. During the camp sessions, the occupational therapists led discussions surrounding emotions and how they affected the body. In the first few weeks of the camp, John explained that when he felt angry or upset, his brain felt like it was jumbled. He also reflected on his aggressive and destructive behaviors and verbalized how those behaviors may be hurting those around him. During these learning opportunities, John began to actively participate in the adaptive response evaluation subprocess. He noted that the existing modes of pushing or hitting others when he became frustrated were ineffective in facilitating friendships. His other existing mode was to become quiet and nonresponsive when presented with challenging tasks. Although he identified that aggressive behaviors were not useful for his interactions with peers, he did not recognize that the existing mode of nonresponsiveness was ineffective. He continued to rely on existing modes and hyperstable adaptive response behaviors when he became upset. It is important to note that becoming nonresponsive may be seen as a protection method during these periods of high stress. As a result, it may be unrealistic to expect that he never display these rigid adaptive response behaviors but rather that they lessen. In the camp, the occupational therapists attempted to facilitate John's adaptive response to reduce the stress of interactions and facilitate his ability to re-engage after stressful events.

Sensory-based and social skill strategies that were discussed in the camp were reviewed with the parents after each day. At the culmination of the camp experience, parents and caregivers were invited to attend a training to review the camp experience and determine how different activities could be incorporated into the children's daily lives to support their generalization of skills to their home environment. After this training, the therapists also had an individual meeting with John's mother. During this meeting, the mother explained her concerns about John engaging in the football season. Together the occupational therapists and the mother problem solved strategies to maximize his success. For example, it was recommended that they explore whether a lineman position would be best for him. The deep pressure provided naturally in the context of this position could serve as a self-regulation strategy. It was also recommended that he wear a skullcap or sweatband to provide deep pressure to his head while also minimizing sweat dripping in his face because he often became overwhelmed by this sensation. Finally, it was recommended that the practice schedule and expectations be clearly described to John. Providing him with this knowledge would increase his ability to adjust his approach to the task.

Approximately 2 months after the camp ended, John's mother updated the occupational therapists on his progress. John was successfully playing a lineman position and participated in all aspects of the practices with intermittent water breaks on the sideline. He had fewer episodes of being upset or overwhelmed during practices. His father and mother were proud of his performance. John adapted to this occupational challenge; both he and his parents deemed his current adaptive responses as successful and satisfying.

ANALYSIS

This case study depicts how occupational therapists can provide opportunities that can empower both a child and their family to be an agent of change in their daily life. In pediatric practice, occupational therapists cannot examine a child in a vacuum. Instead, they must examine how the family structure and interactions can either promote or inhibit a child's success. As evidenced in this case study, John and his mother became partners in his adaptive response generation and evaluation subprocesses. Through this partnership, John learned how to explore new modes and evaluate the success of these modes and behaviors, thus improving his ability to adapt to this occupational challenge. Success in this situation will reinforce his use of new modes and blended behaviors for future occupational challenges.

Case and analysis contributed by Orley A. Templeton, MS, OTD, OTR/L, CAS

Incorporation into the Occupational Environment

Just as the individual's evaluation of the occupational event can result in change (adaptation), evaluation of the same occupational event by the environment has the potential to affect change. It is at the incorporation point, the last step in the process within the environment element of occupational adaptation, that the individual's impact on the occupational environment can be seen. This impact is in the form of influence on the occupational role expectations that are external to the individual. As a result of the individual acting on and within the occupational environment, the role expectations may be subject to change. The expectations may be relaxed in some manner, or conversely, they may be reinforced or intensified. Requirements may be added or subtracted. It is also a possibility that there is no change, and the individual will deal with familiar expectations when encountering or selecting subsequent occupational challenges within that particular context.

Consider the example of an artist who is skilled using pens to draw and markers to add color. The artist desires to expand their use of media and add watercolors to their work. Upon their first attempt, they quickly notice that adding watercolor paint ruins their work; the nonporous paper provides visual and tactile feedback by wrinkling and rejecting the paint. Until the artist discovers a paper suitable for watercolors, they will not experience relative mastery with this new media and may, or may not, doubt their previously accepted role as an accomplished illustrator.

For the therapist to intervene effectively in the client's occupational life, knowledge of the occupational environment in which the client functions is critical. Thinking about this context as physical, social, and cultural in nature gives the therapist a framework for learning about the client's occupational environment and the form, intensity, and character of the expectations that impact a particular client.

TAKE-AWAY MESSAGE

◊ A brief review of the occupational environment and its role in the occupational adaptation process tells us that the occupational environment (a) is composed of physical, social, and cultural influences; (b) has inherent demands for mastery; (c) has external role expectations for the person's performance; (d) involves evaluation of the person's occupational response; and (e) has potential to make changes in external role expectations.

Try It On

In this final Try It On segment, we are going to ask you to identify specific components of the occupational environment related to the same occupational challenge you've been working on, and then reflect on how you and the environment have interacted together.

The following questions will refer you back to your occupational challenge:

Evaluation by the Occupational Environment

How did the occupational environment evaluate your response?

Incorporation into the Occupational Environment

As a result of the environment's evaluation, what alterations would you make, if any, when engaged with the same challenge?

Congratulations on a job well done! Although we have prompted you to "freeze-frame" components of the occupational adaptation process throughout this guide, please keep in mind that this process is dynamic and fluid.

Case 8-1 Worksheet

The Lineman

Name the occupation in context, and then list all aspects of the occupational environment. Consider how each environmental aspect presents expectations and feedback and how the occupational response may change aspects of the occupational environment.

Occupation:				
Environment	**Expectation**	**Feedback**	**Adaptive Response**	**Incorporation**
Physical/Nonhuman				
Social				
Cultural				

Evetts, C. L., & Baxter, M. F. (2024). *Cases and Concepts in Occupational Adaptation: Translating Theory into Action.* SLACK Incorporated.

CHAPTER 9

Assessment and Measures
How Can We Tell Adaptation Is Needed or Occurred?

With contributions from Brooke King, MSOT, OTR/L

*For the reflective occupational therapist,
problem setting is as important as problem solving.*
—Diane Parham (1987, p. 556)

Assessment is a cornerstone of occupational therapy practice. The occupational therapy evaluation guides intervention planning, serving as a road map toward an established destination. A relevant assessment tool will not only help a client realize their progress but will also give occupational therapists the language needed to articulate the value of occupational therapy services to fellow health care practitioners. Furthermore, assessments are one way we justify services to payer sources. All things considered, an important task is choosing assessments that reflect your theoretical orientation, illuminate challenges, and capture progress.

Occupational adaptation requires thoughtful assessment practices, in part because progress may not be captured by typical standardized assessments alone. Remember that the aim of occupational adaptation intervention is not skill mastery but rather adaptation. So, to apply occupational adaptation in practice, it makes sense to use theory-specific resources. Assessment tools specific to occupational adaptation are top down (meaning occupation based) and client centered. That is not to say that an occupational adaptation–focused therapist should totally forgo standardized skill-based assessment tools. Performance skills may be key to how an individual might address an occupational challenge, and supporting body functions contributing to the

Evetts, C. L., & Baxter, M. F. *Cases and Concepts in Occupational Adaptation:
Translating Theory into Action* (pp. 81-88).
DOI: 10.4324/9781003522850-9

adaptation gestalt need to be assessed. Therefore, measuring features such as strength and coordination, visual perception, or executive function remain crucial to a thorough occupational therapy evaluation. Similarly, a thorough knowledge of performance patterns can provide insight when observing dysadaptive behaviors that lead to less-than-desirable levels of relative mastery.

Equally important in the assessment process is to identify client strengths to leverage in responding to occupational challenges. Strengths may include particular body structures and functions or well-developed performance skills, in addition to positive expectations (both internal and externally expressed) that support desire, demand, and press for mastery. The overarching point is that a comprehensive occupational therapy assessment will use a combination of occupational adaptation and standard assessments to capture the person holistically within their meaningful roles and occupational environment(s). This chapter divides the topic of assessment into three components: screening, functional assessment, and measures of relative mastery.

Informal Assessment: Screening and the Occupational Profile

An occupational therapy screen is one of the most informal types of assessment; it is intended as a brief way to investigate whether a potential client could benefit from occupational therapy services. Although strategies to conduct screenings vary between settings, components typically involve chart review, observation and conversation, and dialogue with significant others and other professionals familiar with the individual's functioning. Occupational adaptation theory tells us that transitional periods are most likely to upset the adaptation process. Therefore, when screening individuals, consider their state of transition in recovery between illness or injury and restored health and functioning. Noting difficulty in adapting to challenges may signal a need for further evaluation. Aside from the more obvious transitions, such as a change in performance skills or body functions and structures (e.g., hemiparesis or amputation), transitions may occur at other levels of the occupational therapy domain. For a child with attention-deficit disorder, moving to a new home is an environmental adjustment that could have ripple effects on school performance. Assuming the role of a first-time mother involves a drastic shift in performance patterns. From an occupational lens, transitions could include graduating from or starting a new school, job change or retirement, or driving cessation, just to name a few. Consider collaboration with referral sources to identify transitions relevant to your population that may warrant screening. Using an occupational adaptation lens to identify potential occupational therapy clients shifts the focus from an impairment focus toward holistic assessment.

Occupational Profile

An occupational profile is one of the features of assessment that sets occupational therapy apart from other disciplines. Rather than characterizing an individual by their diagnosis, an occupational therapist who has conducted a thorough occupational profile can characterize their client using more meaningful, occupationally relevant terms (e.g., father, husband, or teacher, as opposed to the more anonymous person with a spinal cord injury). Occupational therapists typically develop an occupational profile during the initial evaluation by learning about the client's occupational experiences, including but not limited to their occupational history, valued occupations, and meaningful roles. This portion of the assessment helps the therapist and client construct an idea of which occupational areas to prioritize and what factors might present challenges on the way to progress. Numerous sources offer guidelines for occupational profile development (American Occupational Therapy Association, 2021; Robinson & Shotwell, 2011). Although the exact structure of the occupational profile will vary between practice settings and clients, the essential elements remain similar. The Canadian Occupational Performance Measure is a well-known tool that has been used with success in practice grounded in occupational adaptation. The Canadian Occupational Performance Measure is an outcome measure that is designed to provide information about a client's self-perception of performance of occupations and satisfaction with them over time (Law & Canadian Association of Occupational Therapists, 1991).

Using an occupational adaptation lens, building the occupational profile is an opportunity to explore factors that will drive the adaptation process. The inquiring therapist should consider environmental factors that demand mastery and personal factors that could spark the desire for mastery. For example, consider how the following situations would shape the direction of goal setting and intervention planning:

- Roles and routines: The importance of meal preparation for a person who thoroughly enjoys cooking meals from scratch compared to a person who goes to a local diner to eat with community members twice a day
- Values and activities of daily living priorities: Differing performance skills needed in self-care activities, such as donning a hijab, wearing pants over a prosthetic leg, applying makeup, or grooming facial hair
- Physical environment: The environmental demands of accessing a group home with ramp entry compared to a walk-up apartment with two flights of stairs
- Occupational participation: The different occupational demands between being a professional musician, a graduate student, a stay-at-home parent, or a retired wage earner

Much like the occupational therapy evaluation itself, the occupational profile should reflect the specific needs and characteristics of the client. The most skillful profile development tends to follow a more natural rhythm rather than

TABLE 9-1

Occupational Adaptation Guide to Practice

OCCUPATIONAL ADAPTATION DATA GATHERING/ASSESSMENT

What are the client's occupational environments and roles? Which role is of primary concern to the client and family?

What occupational performance is expected in the primary occupational environment and role?

What are the physical, social, and cultural features of the primary occupational environment and role?

What is the status of the client's body structures and functions? What performance skills are impacted?

What is the client's level of relative mastery in the primary occupational environment and role?

What is facilitating or limiting relative mastery in the primary occupational environment and role?

What are the client's strengths?

OCCUPATIONAL ADAPTATION PROGRAMMING

What combination of occupational readiness and occupational activity is needed to promote the client's occupational adaptation process?

What help will the client need to assess occupational responses and use the results to affect the occupational adaptation process?

What is the best method to engage the client in the occupational adaptation program?

EVALUATION OF THE OCCUPATIONAL ADAPTATION PROCESS

How is the program affecting the client's occupational adaptation process?
- Which energy level is used most often (primary or secondary)?
- What adaptive response mode is used most often (existing, modified, or new)?
- What is the most common adaptive response behavior (stable, mobile, or blended)?

What outcomes does the client show that reflect change in the occupational adaptation process?
- Self-initiated adaptations?
- Enhanced relative mastery?
- Generalization to novel activities?

What program changes are needed to provide maximum opportunity for occupational adaptation to occur?

Adapted from Schultz, S. & Schkade, J. (1992). Occupational adaptation: Toward a holistic approach for contemporary practice, part 2. *American Journal of Occupational Therapy, 46*(10), 925.

---

the choppy flow of reading standardized questions from a page. Consider the prompts given in this section to be tools in your occupational therapy toolbox. For more ideas about questions to have in mind while constructing an occupational profile, see Table 9-1.

Functional Assessment

Functional assessments refer to assessment tools that are based on occupational performance. As opposed to more biomechanical assessments of discrete skills (e.g., pinch strength measured by a dynamometer), these top-down tools stay true to the profession's value of occupation-based practice. Familiar examples include the Modified Barthel Index, Multiple Errands Test Home Version, and the Kitchen Task Assessment. Functional assessments help establish a baseline level of performance, and using an occupational adaptation perspective, they are also helpful for examining the strategies

an individual uses to adapt to challenges. The Sock Test for Sitting Balance (STSB) was developed with adaptation in mind, and goal attainment scaling (GAS) based on the observation of occupational engagement has been used successfully to measure the impact of intervention on performance, as well as adaptive capacity.

Goal Attainment Scaling

GAS is a method for goal setting that is both standardized and highly individualized. The system has been used since the 1960s as a way of scoring client-centered goals in mental health and rehabilitation fields (Turner-Stokes, 2009). Using GAS, the client and therapist start by identifying a goal and then establishing a realistic set of achievement measures to gauge success. Performance is then scored along a 5-point scale, where −1 is the observed performance at baseline, 0 indicates meeting the expected level of achievement, +2 is far

TABLE 9-2

Martha's Goal Attainment Scale

SCORE	LEVEL OF IMPROVEMENT	SAMPLE GOAL
−2	Much less than expected	Client will complete five knit stitches, given maximal assistance (75%)
−1	Less than expected (baseline)	Client will complete 10 knit stitches, given maximal assistance (50%-75%)
0	Expected outcome	Client will complete 10 neat and even knit stitches, given minimal to moderate assistance (25%-49%)
+1	More than expected	Client will complete two rows of 10 knit stitches with setup assistance and minimal cues (25%)
+2	Much more than expected	Client will complete two rows of 10 knit stitches independently

exceeding expectations, and −2 indicates performance far below the expected outcome. This concept may sound abstract, so before delving in any further, let us explore an example.

Martha is an 80-year-old woman who wants to resume her favorite pastime of knitting after her left hemispheric stroke. Her right hemiparesis is mild, and she presents to an outpatient clinic for rehabilitation. Martha's occupational therapist observes that at baseline she has a rudimentary grasp on the knitting needle in her right hand and can complete knit stitches that are inconsistent in size with maximum (75%) assistance and extended time. Her impaired grasp, in-hand manipulation, and gross motor control impact her ability to perform the intricate motions she typically uses in knitting, and she is very dissatisfied yet highly motivated. The therapist notes in Martha's chart that she was recently discharged from inpatient rehabilitation where she made steady gains. The therapist is optimistic that the client will continue to improve and prioritizes setting goals that are sensitive to change. The client and therapist collaboratively establish GAS, as seen in Table 9-2.

Along the scale, each goal is clearly defined, measurable, and reasonable with the expected intensity and duration of Martha's outpatient therapy participation. Just as importantly, each graded step toward the goal represents a progression collaboratively agreed on by the therapist and the client. For example, in this instance, the GAS illustrates acknowledgment by Martha and her therapist that Martha presently needs maximal assistance, and she is expected to need minimal to moderate assistance before reaching the setup level goal. The fact that goals extend beyond the expected outcome level implies progress along a continuum, which more closely aligns with the dynamic nature of occupational adaptation than a typical static goal might.

Two more qualities make GAS particularly relevant to occupational adaptation: the measure addresses specific occupational goals, and it is sensitive to change. First, GAS personalizes objectives to a client's priorities. Rather than searching for a (likely nonexistent or minimally relevant) measure that relates to personal occupational pursuits, such as knitting, preparing meals with an air fryer, fly-fishing, or guitar playing, GAS provides a structured approach to occupation-based goal setting. Because the client is actively involved in determining appropriate progression, the client and therapist essentially co-construct the goals for treatment. Second, GAS facilitates the development of goals that are not only meaningful to the client but also sensitive to change.

For contrast, picture Martha's therapist using the Nine-Hole Peg Test as a measurement of her fine motor coordination as related to knitting. The resulting score can be compared to age-related averages; however, this does not give insight into Martha's actual knitting performance. Furthermore, Martha can see improvement in her knitting capabilities (whether through the use of adaptive strategies or improved motor control), thereby maintaining her desire to meet the demands of knitting. In contrast, the change in a Nine-Hole Peg Test score may be minimal and even non-meaningful to Martha, artificially capping her progress. Instances like this illustrate how one-dimensional goals may not capture the subtle functional improvement and adaptive gains that are so impactful to clients' lives.

Another example of using GAS in the context of a program guided by occupational adaptation was described for women with intellectual and developmental disabilities who were incarcerated (Stelter & Evetts, 2020). A bank of possible goals was established to align with the occupational therapy program designed to help women prepare for release from prison. The bank included goals for social participation,

TABLE 9-3
Example From a Goal Attainment Scale Bank

GOAL AREA	EMOTIONAL REGULATION AND COPING			
Persists through challenges	Independently persists through challenges	Persists through challenges with indirect cue or modeling	Persists through challenges with direct verbal cue	Persists through a portion of a challenge with direct verbal cue
Expected levels of outcome	2	1	0	−1

The occupational therapist selects a goal and sets the scale with −1 at the baseline observation. (Adapted from Stelter, L. [2018]. *The impact of an occupation-based program for incarcerated women with intellectual and developmental disabilities* [Doctoral dissertation, Texas Woman's University]. ProQuest Dissertations Publishing [No. 13846793].)

emotion regulation and coping, problem solving, decision making, and more. The on-site occupational therapist then selected a goal for each participant based on observation of functioning in the context of meaningful activity. Table 9-3 provides an example of a client in a cooking group who was observed initially trying to peel a carrot but gave up even with encouragement. In this case, the goal (0) was set for her to persist with direct verbal cues.

Sock Test for Sitting Balance

Much the same way that a measure such as the Nine-Hole Peg Test may not directly correlate with occupational performance, balance assessments often lack a functional component. The STSB is a functional sitting balance assessment that may be especially useful for occupational therapists in an acute care setting because of its quick and easy administration and efficient use of readily available supplies. To administer the assessment, a therapist needs a stopwatch and a pair of hospital socks with grip soles. Hospital socks with grip soles are available as a standard issue for most hospital clients and are part of a fall prevention tool across many hospital settings.

Administration

To administer the STSB, the therapist sits across from the client who is sitting unsupported on the edge of a hospital bed or chair. The therapist asks the client to don and doff a pair of hospital socks and times the client in the performance of the task. The client can use whatever strategy for donning and doffing the socks they are comfortable with, including crossed leg or bending down. The average time for donning and doffing socks is between 19 and 22 seconds. Furthermore, the average time to don and doff does not depend on the strategy used.

Before administering the STSB, the therapist documents possible impairments in vision, fine motor, cognition, and so on. Then, during the administration, the therapist observes the client's movement patterns, problem-solving tactics, and notable compensations, thereby gaining insight into adaptive strategies and patterns during this functional task that requires dynamic sitting balance (Franc et al., 2020).

Scores on the assessment are correlated with other measures of balance and function, including the Kansas University Sitting and Standing Balance Scales, as well as the Functional Independence Measure chair transfer subscore. Specifically, a longer time to complete the STSB correlates with lower transfer scores and a lower balance rating on the Functional Independence Measure (Franc et al., 2020). By incorporating a functional task that requires dynamic sitting balance and accommodates for the variety of ways that individuals naturally perform donning and doffing socks, the STSB is an occupation-based alternative to timed balance tests (Nicholson, 2012; Parker, 2011). The STSB also considers relative mastery in that task completion can be accomplished in a variety of ways and the adaptive patterns of task completion are considered. An increased time is not a "fail" in the STSB; rather, it can be used as a measure of progress or regression if time improves or deteriorates on repeated administrations. Finally, as mentioned previously, the STSB can be administered with limited materials and in a short amount of time, making it an easy way to incorporate occupational adaptation into hospital-based practice.

Measures of Relative Mastery

In occupational adaptation, relative mastery is the lens through which occupational performance is evaluated. Schkade and Schultz (1992) explain this as follows:

Relative mastery is the extent to which the person experiences the occupational response as efficient (use of time and energy), effective (production of the desired result), and satisfying to self and society; that is, it is pleasing not only to the self but also to relevant others as agents of the occupational environment. (p. 835)

For occupational therapists, the concept of relative mastery is useful in performing nuanced assessments. Rather than scoring a client on the metrics of their performance alone, relative mastery considers the adaptation strategies a person uses, as well as the role of environmental feedback. The therapist is looking for responses that balance efficiency, effectiveness, and satisfaction to self and others. Relative mastery can be integrated into one's occupational therapy practice with both informal and standardized approaches.

Informal Application

When applying occupational adaptation principles, relative mastery serves as a compass pointing toward client-centered practice. Although traditional occupational therapy practices tend to focus on maximizing client independence, the outcomes of occupational adaptation intervention may look different when evaluated through the lens of relative mastery. As an example, picture a man who seriously struggles to don his shoes using adaptive equipment after a posterior total hip replacement. Perhaps he makes statements like, "When I get home, my wife will be happy to put my shoes on for me." In a traditional frame of reference that emphasizes activities of daily living independence, therapists may gravitate toward encouraging the client to continue attempting to use the equipment despite the increased time and frustration he experiences. Understandably, encouraging independence may reflect institutional principles (such as facility rankings based on the level of improved activities of daily living scores) or may be foundational to successful discharge planning (e.g., if the client lives alone).

However, to consider another perspective, let us picture the client's options using relative mastery as a guide. Using adaptive equipment to don his shoes uses extensive time and energy; this strategy is not efficient for him. When he dons his shoes, he struggles to pull up the tongue of the shoe, and his sock feels askew; this strategy does not feel effective. Furthermore, he does not place high value on donning his own shoes, offering the solution that his wife dons his shoes (and thus illustrating that this option might be acceptable to both him and his partner). In this scenario, a more masterful response may in fact be for the client and his wife to collaborate in footwear management. This individual's supportive social environment (characterized by his wife) offers the opportunity for an adaptive response that is efficient, effective, and satisfactory to himself and others (his wife and perhaps the therapy team as well).

To approach relative mastery from another angle, the concept can be used as a tool to help a client evaluate their options and assess their progress. Reflective questions such as "How satisfied are you with the time this strategy takes?" or "Do you feel content with your performance?" bring attention to the client's experience of relative mastery and set the stage for adaptive response generation. In some instances, a therapist may notice that a client is quite satisfied with a method of performing a task even though the strategy appears unconventional to the therapist. Professional judgment aids the therapist in determining when to intervene as an agent of the environment to bring attention to safety concerns. Regardless, a skilled clinician will empower clients to adapt in ways that feel most efficient, effective, and satisfactory to themselves.

A simple way to document self-report of relative mastery is to ask the client to rate their level of efficiency on a scale of 1 to 5, with 1 representing not at all efficient and 5 being completely efficient. Use the same 5-point scale for ratings of effectiveness, satisfaction to self, and satisfaction to others. Add the four scales, and the sum provides an overall rating of relative mastery on a scale of 4 (*very low*) to 20 (*very high*). Upon repeated measures, a change in any of the four scales will impact the total score; it will be important to note which individual scales rise or fall in determining the success of intervention. For example, it may be that as some scales improve, others may drop until the client establishes a balance of meeting internal and external expectations.

Occupational therapists and researchers have been successful in adapting the informal use of relative mastery to meet the needs of specific client populations. For example, when prompting adults with intellectual disabilities to assess relative mastery, a visual 3-point scale was devised for efficiency ("How smooth did my work go?"), effectiveness ("How good was my work?"), and satisfaction ("How do I feel about my work?") using common symbols and simple words on a poster (Stelter, 2018). The goal is not to obtain a particular score but to prompt individuals to self-reflect so that adaptive capacity can grow.

Standardized: Relative Mastery Measurement Scale

A more formal and quantitative way to assess a client's experience of relative mastery is with the Relative Mastery Measurement Scale (RMMS). This assessment evaluates relative mastery using an occupational adaptation frame of reference, and it serves as one of the primary assessment tools developed specifically to complement occupational adaptation (Krusen & George-Paschal, 2018). The RMMS consists of 12 prompts that relate to aspects of relative mastery. The client is asked to think about a specific activity they have just completed and then to state whether they agree or disagree with each statement based on their self-assessment. Prompts alternate between positive and negative wording (e.g., "I am very pleased with my performance of this task" and "I failed to complete all steps of the task"; George et al., 2004, p. 102). Scores range from 0 to 12, with a score of 5 or below indicating a perception of poor relative mastery (George et al., 2004). Statistical analysis of the measure demonstrates the RMMS is sensitive to change, reliable, and useful in inpatient rehabilitation, academia, and mental health settings (George et al., 2004; George-Paschal & Bowen, 2019; Krusen & George-Paschal, 2018).

Aside from providing objective data points to measure progress, the RMMS is valuable in stimulating self-evaluation of performance. Central to occupational adaptation is the idea that the client's adaptation drives progress. In administering the RMMS, the therapist acts as an agent of the environment, presenting an external cue (the RMMS prompts) to facilitate self-assessment as the client reflects on their experience of relative mastery in a certain task.

Connecting Assessment to Intervention: The Occupational Adaptation Practice Guide

So far, this chapter has addressed multiple formal and informal strategies to integrate occupational adaptation principles into assessment. The final tool addressed in this chapter combines occupational adaptation principles into a guide for assessment and treatment.

Aptly named, the Occupational Adaptation Practice Guide (OAPG) is a tool that guides evaluation and intervention planning. It is designed to facilitate applying occupational adaptation in daily occupational therapy practice. The OAPG consists of three structured sections: data gathering, person and environment analysis, and program planning (Boone & George-Paschal, 2017). Open-ended prompts enable cooperation between the client and practitioner in generating goals, identifying relevant strengths and barriers, and planning intervention (Boone & George-Paschal, 2017). In fact, the process touches on adaptive response generation as clients reflect on their goals and strategies to reach them. Because of its open-ended nature, the tool can be applied across a range of populations; of note, practitioners have successfully used the OAPG in inpatient rehabilitation and emerging practice areas (Boone & George-Paschal, 2017; George-Paschal & Bowen, 2019; Green et al., 2021).

As a whole, the OAPG is an efficient tool to guide therapists in using theory in a clear, comprehensive way. Similar to the Canadian Occupational Performance Measure, the OAPG walks the therapist and client through step-by-step guidance to collaboratively engage in the assessment process. Therefore, from the outset, the client identifies relevant occupational goals and is guided through applying a holistic lens to reflect on the environmental and personal demands that may impact their performance. Therapists who used the measure reflected that the OAPG was helpful for efficiently bringing together theory and intervention planning (Boone & George-Paschal, 2017). For an even more holistic occupational adaptation application, the OAPG can be used in conjunction with the RMMS for quantitative measurement.

FUTURE RESEARCH

Assessment tools to support the use of occupational adaptation in practice are still being developed. Preliminary evidence is documented in case studies and unpublished scholarly work, especially out of Texas Woman's University. Emerging assessment tools include the Assessment of Relative Mastery in Occupational Roles (Stelter & Whisner, 2007) and the Guided Occupational Exploration (Evetts, n.d.), which provide novel ways to integrate occupational adaptation into practice but remain untested on a large scale. Occupational adaptation is in an exciting stage in which there remains opportunity to trial, refine, and innovate assessments that tap into the essence of adaptation and the subtleties of occupation-based practice.

TAKE-AWAY MESSAGES

◊ Occupational adaptation principles can be integrated throughout the assessment process, from occupational profile development to goal setting and standardized measurement.

◊ GAS is a way to document change in observed performance of meaningful occupation.

◊ The STSB is an occupation-based tool for assessing client performance from an occupational adaptation perspective.

◊ The RMMS is a self-evaluation tool that is also helpful in facilitating client insight into their experience of relative mastery.

◊ The OAPG facilitates applying theory to practice with structured steps that are highly collaborative between the client and the therapist.

References

American Occupational Therapy Association. (2021). Improve your documentation and quality of care with AOTA's updated occupational profile template. *American Journal of Occupational Therapy, 75*, 7502420010. https://doi.org/10.5014/ajot.2021.752001

Boone, A. E., & George-Paschal, L. A. (2017). Feasibility testing of the Occupational Adaptation Practice Guide. *British Journal of Occupational Therapy, 80*(6), 368-374. https://doi.org/10.1177/0308022616688018

Evetts, C. (n.d.). *Guided occupational exploration.* Unpublished manuscript, Department of Occupational Therapy, Texas Woman's University.

Franc, I. A., Baxter, M. F., Mitchell, K., Neville, M., & Chang, P.-F. (2020). Validity of the Sock Test for Sitting Balance: A functional sitting balance assessment. *OTJR: Occupation, Participation and Health, 40*(3), 159-165. https://doi.org/10.1177%2F1539449220905807

George, L. A., Schkade, J. K., & Ishee, J. H. (2004). Content validity of the Relative Mastery Measurement Scale: A measure of occupational adaptation. *OTJR: Occupation, Participation and Health, 24*(3), 92-102. https://doi.org/10.1177/153944920402400303

George-Paschal, L., & Bowen, M. R. (2019). Outcomes of a mentoring program based on occupational adaptation for participants in a juvenile drug court program. *Occupational Therapy in Mental Health, 35*(3), 262-286. https://doi.org/10.1080/0164212X.2019.1601605

Green, J., George-Paschal, L., Harmon, T., Archibald-Hill, M., Poff, A., & Womack, B. K. (2021). Assessing the usability and reliability of the Occupational Adaptation Practice Guide in an adult inpatient rehabilitation setting [Poster]. *American Journal of Occupational Therapy, 75*(Suppl. 2), 7512500029. https://doi.org/10.5014/ajot.2021.75S2-PO29

Krusen, N., & George-Paschal, L. (2018). Relative Mastery Measurement Scale as an effective, profession-specific, theoretically founded learning outcome measure. *American Journal of Occupational Therapy, 74*(4 Suppl. 1), 72115000671. https://doi.org/10.5014/ajot.2018.72S1-PO8006

Law, M., & Canadian Association of Occupational Therapists. (1991). *Canadian Occupational Performance Measure.* CAOT Publications ACE.

Nicholson, J. D. (2012). *Measuring sock donning and doffing in a normal population* (Unpublished master's thesis). Texas Woman's University.

Parham, D. (1987). Toward professionalism: The reflective therapist. *American Journal of Occupational Therapy, 41*(9), 555-561. https://doi.org/10.5014/ajot.41.9.555

Parker, B. S. (2011). *Development and use of the sock test in acute care rehabilitation* (Unpublished master's thesis). Texas Woman's University.

Robinson, K. T., & Shotwell, M. (2011). Evaluation of the acute care patient. In H. Smith-Gabai (Ed.), *Occupational therapy in acute care* (pp. 1-29). AOTA Press.

Schkade, J. K., & Schultz, S. (1992) Occupational adaptation: Toward a holistic approach for contemporary practice, part 1. *American Journal of Occupational Therapy, 46*(9), 829-837. https://doi.org/10.5014/ajot.46.9.829

Stelter, L. (2018). *The impact of an occupation-based program for incarcerated women with intellectual and developmental disabilities* (Doctoral dissertation, Texas Woman's University). ProQuest Dissertations Publishing (No. 13846793).

Stelter, L. D., & Evetts, C. L. (2020). Effect of an occupation-based program for women with intellectual and developmental disabilities who are incarcerated. *Annals of International Occupational Therapy, 3*(4), 175-184. https://doi.org/10.3928/24761222-20190910-01

Stelter, L., & Whisner, S. M. (2007). Building responsibility for self through meaningful roles: Occupational adaptation theory applied in forensic psychiatry. *Occupational Therapy in Mental Health, 23*(1), 69-84. https://doi.org/10.1300/J004v23n01_05

Turner-Stokes, L. (2009). Goal attainment scaling (GAS) in rehabilitation: A practice guide. *Clinical Rehabilitation, 23*(4), 362-370. https://doi.org/10.1177/0269215508101742

CHAPTER 10

Intervention Tools, Therapist as Agent of the Environment, Client as Agent of Change

What Does the Therapist Do?

Go to the people
Work with them
Learn from them
Respect them
Start with what they know

Build with what they have.
And when the work is done
The task accomplished
The people will say,
"We have done this ourselves."

—Lao Tsu

Intervention

In occupational therapy practice, we often describe the strategies therapists use with their clients as "tools." The occupational therapist has several therapeutic tools that are applicable regardless of the frame of reference guiding the therapist's thinking. The therapist who practices from an occupational adaptation perspective uses those familiar strategies, as well as some that are more theory specific. There are four core therapeutic tools recommended for use in occupational adaptation practice:

1. Practitioner is the agent of the occupational environment.

2. Practitioner incorporates principles of therapeutic use of self.

3. Practitioner uses occupation to promote adaptiveness.

4. Client is the agent of change (Schultz, 2014, p. 539).

Let us talk first about three of the customary tools that every therapist has learned, and then we will talk more specifically about how the therapist functions from an occupational adaptation point of view.

Evetts, C. L., & Baxter, M. F. *Cases and Concepts in Occupational Adaptation:*
Translating Theory into Action (pp. 89-98).
DOI: 10.4324/9781003522850-10

Familiar Intervention Tools

Knowledge base is the first obviously important tool for any intervention—knowledge of the person–system structures and how they interrelate and function in the service of occupation. The therapist must understand how dysfunction in these interrelated structures affects dysfunction in occupational performance. This is where a thorough understanding of activity analysis comes into play. In other words, what are the motor, process, and interaction skill requirements of occupational performance in general? This knowledge tool is the basis from which you apply general knowledge to particular clients in specific instances.

Therapeutic bag of tricks is a second important tool. This includes various evaluations, intervention techniques, knowledge of assistive aids and technologies, ability to identify the need for environmental modifications, and additional ways to make therapeutic use of available tools and materials (Bachman, 2016). The therapist must know whether or when it is appropriate to use these various skill sets. In her distinguished scholar lecture to the American Occupational Therapy Association assembly in 2002, Dr. Mary C. Law (2002) cautioned that it is easier to teach skills than to facilitate participation and foster resilience. Increasing adaptive capacity will go much further in helping someone become a functional person than teaching them a list of skills. Grejo (2017) asserted that "The occupational therapist must resist using direct teaching as a therapeutic tool" (p. 301).

In the 2013 Eleanor Clarke Slagle lecture, Dr. Glen Gillen issued a strong call to put occupation back into occupational therapy, with a reminder that engagement in true occupation is not only our roots, but it is also our hope for success in the future. To reinforce the distinct value of occupational therapy, we need to embrace occupation as our primary tool for assessment and intervention (Gillen, 2013). Five years later in the 2018 Eleanor Clarke Slagle lecture, Dr. Gordon Giles reinforced the need for strengthening the profession through the application of occupation-based practice. "Engaging the client in meaningful activity is the art and science of occupational therapy, and it will never be superseded by technological innovation because true creativity and genuine empathy cannot be mechanized" (Giles, 2018, p. 13).

Therapeutic use of self is an extremely important tool. In other words, as a therapist, you need the ability to position yourself physically, cognitively, and psychosocially to facilitate your client's progress. You must be able to facilitate your client's progress through your carefully developed intervention plan. You must also be positioned to respond to unplanned and unexpected events in such a way as to be therapeutic. You must be attuned to information the client provides that was not a part of your assessment but surfaced naturally during the course of therapeutic interactions.

In her 2011 Eleanor Clarke Slagle lecture, Dr. Betty Abreu provided six guiding questions inferred by clients that can enhance therapeutic relationship using empathy:

1. How do others like me cope and adapt?
2. Are you sure you want to enter my world?
3. How can you better understand our language?
4. What is my hope and strength?
5. How can I problem solve more effectively?
6. Can we have fun today? (Abreu, 2011, p. 628)

The therapist who heeds these unspoken but inferred questions is reminded to listen carefully to the client's desires and the demands they feel from their occupational environments. When we fully understand their story, we are more likely to be in a position to facilitate success as our clients respond to occupational challenges in their press for mastery.

For the therapist who wishes to practice from an occupational adaptation perspective, the three tools previously described are required. Remember that occupational adaptation theory was developed to "name and frame what good therapists do" (J. Schkade, personal communication, March 30, 1993). The following case of The Artist (Case 10-1) is an example of how a good therapist came to recognize how her intervention could be explained by occupational adaptation theory, even though at the time, she was simply operating with familiar intervention tools. Now that she has gained awareness of what created the significant positive transition for her client, she can be more intentional in facilitating adaptive responses with others.

The familiar tools for occupational therapy practice, including a solid knowledge base, skillful application of strategies (the bag of tricks), and therapeutic use of self, are essential to effective intervention. To facilitate adaptive capacity that will generalize beyond the current disruption in functioning, a few additional tools are necessary.

Occupational Adaptation Reasoning Skills

An understanding of the concepts and their relationships (i.e., how the occupational adaptation process works) is necessary. Occupational adaptation is not a technique or a set of techniques. It is a way of thinking about your client and about how you approach your task as a therapist. The focus of intervention is always on the client and a client-selected occupational role. In his 1999 Eleanor Clarke Slagle lecture, Dr. Charles Christiansen (1999) discussed the idea that what people do (their occupations) contributes significantly to their identity.

CASE 10-1

The Artist

When Jack came to inpatient rehabilitation, his outlook was bleak. He presented to the hospital with serious osteomyelitis, a spinal cord injury, and a social situation complicated by homelessness and heroin addiction. As Jack and I discussed his occupational profile and set goals, his focus was less on physical function and more on lifestyle changes that could support his recovery from drug addiction.

Sustaining a spinal cord injury was a life-altering event that sparked Jack's desire to discontinue using heroin. The combination of his internal drive for mastery and environmental factors (including the hospital setting, therapists, and peers) generated a sustained press for mastery that propelled him to actively engage in his recovery. Through therapeutic interviews, Jack and I identified that his occupational challenge was to use healthy strategies to handle stress and to identify alternative occupations to fill his time.

A barrier to Jack's adaptation was the extensive effort required to break out of his deeply ingrained habits (existing adaptive response mode, rigid adaptive response behavior). When explicitly discussing community programs, meditation strategies, and potential occupational outlets, Jack became frustrated and said he felt overwhelmed. During a particularly meaningful intervention session that departed from our direct focus on his recovery, I structured for Jack an activity of designing and assembling his own leather-bound sketchbook. Jack was completely engrossed in the task, demonstrating a level of focus I had not yet seen from him. For the duration of his participation, he appeared calm and focused. Jack decided that artistically working with his hands was his preferred strategy to meet his occupational challenge of replacing his addictive habits with meaningful activity. In fact, months after Jack was discharged from rehab, he returned to the hospital with his sketchbook to share that he had stayed sober for 8 months, a feat he credited to his renewed engagement in creating art.

ANALYSIS

In an inpatient rehabilitation setting, environmental factors such as strict substance control and visitor restrictions eliminated Jack's access to illicit substances. Furthermore, taking a narrow approach to address only the occupational habit of substance use had been ineffective for him in the past. As George-Paschal and Bowen (2019) explained, adults with a criminal offender history may benefit from participating in interventions framed by occupational adaptation. "The cycle of continuing to make the same mistakes with the same negative outcomes may have resulted from having fewer strategies … leading to a failure to abandon ineffective strategies" (p. 266). Although I did not realize it at the time, my intervention with Jack facilitated an adaptive response, particularly by targeting his adaptation energy and adaptive modes. Jack engaged in adaptive response generation as he shifted to new adaptive response modes, providing opportunities to shift from primary to secondary energy and ultimately producing an adaptive response that impacted his occupational role as an artist.

At the time, I lacked the vocabulary for what I witnessed; however, in retrospect, it is apparent that Jack had shifted from using primary to secondary energy. Although he actively focused on this task, he was subconsciously using secondary energy to solve the underlying issue we had been addressing for weeks. The sketchbook, which I had envisioned as a meaningful way to engage his hands, tapped into a deeper state of mind and made clear a solution that had been present all along.

Collaborating with Jack and structuring opportunities for successful participation were effective in fostering an adaptive occupational response. Initially, I presented him with concrete strategies, which were ultimately ineffectual (although occupational readiness is potentially helpful). Later, by structuring opportunities for Jack to feel successful and tap into secondary energy, he began genuinely engaging in an adaptive process. The fact that Jack sustained his new response behaviors for months outside the hospital environment demonstrated the value of occupational therapy services in nurturing an individual's ability to adapt to their circumstances in new and meaningful ways.

Case and analysis contributed by Brooke King, MSOT, OTR/L

Therapy becomes identity building when therapists provide environments that help persons explore possible selves and achieve success in tasks that are instrumental to identities they strive to achieve, and when it enables them to validate the identities that they have worked hard to achieve in the past. (p. 555)

As applied to occupational adaptation, focusing intervention on occupational roles taps into a person's identity, to the very core of their being. When a person has lost their sense of purpose or identity, aiming to improve occupational role performance keeps intervention occupation focused, occupation based, and distinct as occupational therapy.

Concrete guidelines for intervention grounded in the theory are offered by Cole and Tufano (2008), who identified nine strategies based on occupational adaptation concepts:

1. Learn about the client's expectations of their identified occupational role.
2. Facilitate participation in meaningful social interaction.
3. Use a strengths-based approach for promoting adaptive capacity.
4. Enable active participation in producing meaningful outcomes.
5. Prompt conscious assessment of relative mastery.
6. Plan for both occupational readiness and occupational engagement.
7. Provide direct feedback related to adaptive responses.
8. Prompt client to identify alternative responses when relative mastery is not achieved.
9. Use the Occupational Adaptation Practice Guide to promote self-awareness of patterns of strengths and challenges. (pp. 112-113)

Obviously, such a brief summary cannot be applied effectively without a thorough knowledge of the underlying theory; the "why" (theory) guides the when, what, and how of therapeutic intervention for each client.

Occupational adaptation tells you what questions to ask, not "what to do." In his 2018 Eleanor Clarke Slagle lecture, Dr. Gordon Giles (2018) asserted the following:

… people remember what they think, not what you tell them. So if you are telling someone that they should do X, Y, and Z, and they are thinking that you are a fool, then what they will remember is that you are a fool. (p. 7)

The point is not that you may appear foolish; the point is that people are more likely to remember and adopt solutions (adaptations) that they figure out for themselves, so do not attempt to impress others with your ability to come up with a great solution. Your job is to "know the answer, [but] ask the question" (S. Schultz, personal communication, March 30, 1993).

The general questions presented in Table 9-1 (refer to Chapter 9) do not change from client to client. However, the answers will be very different for each individual. Once the client provides you with answers, then you begin to plan your intervention using the client-selected occupational role(s). Remember that dysfunction is always relative to the occupational role. If you have identified a deficit in the body structures, functions, or even a skill set that does not relate to the occupational role, do not get stuck there. This should not be the focus for therapy. Likewise, if a particular deficit (e.g., range of motion limitation) does not interfere with the occupational performance that the client has selected, do not get stuck here either. Similarly, the same deficit may impact occupational performance differently from one client to the other. One size does not fit all in this case. A pianist and a forklift operator with the "same" deficit in finger mobility have different therapeutic needs. Therefore, when an identified deficit does interfere with occupational performance and role participation, use whatever therapeutic tools are appropriate to limit interference and support function in the identified occupational role.

A collaborative relationship with the client is essential in occupational adaptation practice. Your goal is that the client will serve as their own change agent. Your task is not to take away that function from the client. This is very important because in occupational adaptation you are always trying to facilitate the client's internal adaptation capabilities. If you do not let the client exercise their own agency, how can you expect the client's internal adaptation capabilities to be strengthened? The answer is a no-brainer; you cannot.

Nevertheless, you still have a very important role to play. Your task is to serve as the agent of the environment in which the client's occupational role is carried out. In other words, you have to set the stage for the client to carry out their role-related tasks just as the environment does when the client is in their usual surroundings or context.

Practitioner as Agent of the Occupational Environment

What exactly does it mean to be the "agent of the occupational environment?" First, you have to learn what the demands of that environment are relative to the occupational role. (Remember the demand for mastery and the occupational role expectations?) Very often, these demands and expectations are something with which you may not be familiar. There may be economic influences, social influences, cultural influences, family influences, and more that determine how the client is expected to perform. You must enter a collaborative therapeutic relationship and be willing to place yourself in the role of "learner" and allow the client to become the "teacher." Otherwise, how can you possibly plan relevant intervention? In addition, allowing the client to teach you helps build therapeutic rapport and is a wonderful empowerment tool in permitting the client to serve as a self-changing agent.

> Doing by the patient . . . rather than doing to the patient—that's really justice a lot of times. You know, I assert to my students, that sometimes the things that we do and the things that we say in therapy are actually occupational justice inhibiting, or inadvertently promoting injustice, when making the decision for our patients. Always *telling* the patients what they need to do, rather than *discovering* what they should be doing, we're inadvertently sort of promoting some marginalization and some injustices there. (L. Grejo, personal communication, April 7, 2019)

Remember, a strong tenet in occupational therapy is learn by doing. Doing is a much better reinforcement for learning or remembering than simply receiving instruction. Often, students and therapists are initially confused by the admonition to resist teaching the client as part of therapy. Consider the following: there are many ways to promote learning that do not involve direct instruction.

Dr. Patricia Fingerhut (an occupational therapist, professor, and occupational adaptation scholar), in describing her work with children, revealed her belief that being "playfully obstructive" can elicit an adaptive response (personal communication, October 2020). Within an established therapeutic relationship, playfully creating just-right challenges in real time can tap into internal (desire) and external (demand) motivation and elicit a press for mastery.

Dr. Maralynne Mitcham's 2014 Eleanor Clarke Slagle lecture, "Education as Engine," offered sound advice that we can relate to facilitating adaptive responses. Yes, when operating under an occupational adaptation perspective, direct teaching is discouraged. However, learning is not dependent on teacher input. Learning is an internal process in the same way that adaptation is an internal process. Dr. Mitcham (2014) reminded us of the following important aspects of learning that can occur in the context of occupational therapy:

- Individuals learn best through making sense and meaning of their experiences over time.
- Learning is best constructed in a variety of contents.
- The most authentic context will offer the most meaningful learning.
- Individuals have to actively participate and engage with the challenges presented. (p. 641)

Thus, acting as an agent of the environment to set up engaging role-related occupational challenges provides clients with opportunities to learn by doing in the context of their everyday living, whether simulated or in real time.

Dr. Laurie Stelter, an occupational therapy educator and occupational adaptation scholar, developed a set of "therapeutic ingredients" that can be modified for specific clients (whether individuals, groups, or populations). These ingredients are embedded in therapeutic programs to provide opportunities for role-related participation and production of adaptive responses to everyday challenges. Based on earlier work with men with mental illness who were incarcerated (Stelter & Whisner, 2007), a program was designed specifically for women with intellectual and developmental disorders and mental illness who were incarcerated (Stelter & Evetts, 2020). The following list is modified to provide general guidelines. When operating a practice based on occupational adaptation, the therapist intentionally provides opportunities to (a) select, plan, and execute meaningful activity and evaluate task performance; (b) create tangible products or intangible but recognizable outcomes; (c) engage in graded, just-right occupational challenges; (d) receive direct or indirect verbal or physical assistance only as necessary; (e) receive objective, nonjudgmental feedback; (f) participate in novel tasks or contexts; (g) engage in a positive social environment; and (h) experience self in an occupational role that is personally satisfying.

Each of these therapeutic ingredients is grounded in the concepts of occupational adaptation theory. As a way to check your understanding, can you come up with a "why" statement for each of the ingredients? Use the Therapeutic Ingredients worksheet at the end of this chapter, and check your responses against the answer key in Appendix B.

The blend of knowledge base, bag of tricks, therapeutic use of self, understanding of occupational adaptation concepts, engaging in a collaborative relationship, and acting as an agent of the occupational environment by knowing what questions to ask and providing therapeutic ingredients come together to promote the client's adaptive capacity. The case of The Pianist (Case 10-2) provides an example of how a therapist used a wide variety of her therapeutic skills to engage the client in an intervention approach that was consistent with occupational adaptation principles.

The Pianist case demonstrates how a skillful therapist used necessary tools from an occupational adaptation perspective as follows:

- She saw indications that the client still desired mastery (inferred from her appearance).
- She identified an occupational role that was meaningful (pianist).
- She served as the agent of the occupational environment (set the stage for the client to engage in her occupation).
- Most importantly, she collaborated with the client, allowing the client to become her own agent of change (identifying strategies the client could use to create piano-playing opportunities).

The therapist facilitated adaptiveness in the client that would enhance her ability to engage in her preferred occupation, and her newly awakened desire for mastery generalized such that she began participating in therapeutic groups. The Woodworker (Case 10-3) demonstrates how another therapist practicing from an occupational adaptation perspective approached intervention.

CASE 10-2

The Pianist

Mrs. Evans was a patient in an acute psychiatric unit with a diagnosis of schizophrenia. She had been hospitalized on many occasions. A review of her chart indicated that she had very limited social interaction and refused most groups. The occupational therapy intern went to the patient's room to interview her. She found Mrs. Evans in a dark room with the lights off, curtains closed, and the bedcovers pulled over her head. Mrs. Evans was uneasy about the therapist but agreed to answer a few questions. After about 4 minutes, Mrs. Evans "dismissed" the therapist but was rather polite.

During the short interview, the therapist noted that Mrs. Evans had long painted fingernails with chipped polish, dyed jet-black hair, and considerable makeup. The therapist had limited information from the interview itself, but her observations led her to believe that appearance was important to Mrs. Evans. The therapist located shades of fingernail polish from various staff members and returned to Mrs. Evans' room, inquiring if she would like to redo her nails. Mrs. Evans was interested but did not want to go to the dayroom to do it. However, she did so.

Mrs. Evans opened up to the therapist as she painted her nails, with the assistance of the therapist. During this time, Mrs. Evans revealed that she had studied art and music in college and taught piano for many years. She had four children. She had grown up on a farm where she had developed a love of horseback riding. However, it had been a number of years since she had engaged in the activities she enjoyed.

Mrs. Evans lived in an assisted living environment where there was no longer a piano available. Together, Mrs. Evans and the therapist worked on identifying places in the community where she could have access to a piano. Mrs. Evans attended Alcoholics Anonymous meetings weekly at a church where there was a piano. The therapist helped Mrs. Evans identify the appropriate person from whom to gain permission to use the piano and how he might be contacted. Mrs. Evans also identified other places in the community where she could try to locate a piano.

The therapist gained permission to take Mrs. Evans off the unit to a location in the hospital where there was a piano. When she sat down to play, staff members from offices along the hallway came out to see who was playing so beautifully. Later, the therapist brought music books and sheet music for Mrs. Evans to select to take home. She was excited about being able to play again.

Mrs. Evans also started coming to the task group and began participating in groups that were addressing other goals.

Case contributed by Catherine Evich Johnson, OTS

The Woodworker case is a good example of how an occupational therapist practicing from occupational adaptation "tuned in" to the information regarding personally meaningful occupation provided by her client. She then capitalized on that information to achieve a successful therapeutic outcome. It also demonstrates how in the "physical dysfunction" setting, it was her attention to the heavy psychosocial content of his communication that led to his engagement in intervention (Bachman, 2016). She placed him in a situation in which he was the "expert" by allowing him to teach her about the Dremel (Bosch Power Tools) and permitting him to critique her technique. She also exercised patience and did not give up due to his initial reluctance and earlier refusals.

This skillful therapist used the principles discussed in this chapter—knowledge base, techniques, therapeutic use of self, understanding of occupational adaptation, asking therapeutically appropriate questions, and engaging Mr. Robinson in a collaborative relationship with her. When the therapist takes this approach, the results can meet the needs of all parties concerned in the rehabilitation effort. The goals of the referring physician were met; the facility's need to provide effective services was met; and, most importantly, Mr. Robinson's need to be rehabilitated in a therapeutic climate where his views, values, and talent were respected was met. The outcome was satisfying to both the client and the therapist.

The case of The New Resident (Case 10-4) is an example of a therapist who saw beyond her client's deficits to a broader issue of occupational justice. In this case, the therapist acted as an agent of the client's environment to enable occupations that had been previously dismissed or denied.

CASE 10-3

The Woodworker

Mr. Robinson was a 62-year-old man hospitalized for rehabilitation secondary to deconditioning. The deconditioning was the result of a complex medical history that included hypertension, a myocardial infarction, and a quadruple arterial bypass procedure.

Before the initial assessment by an occupational therapist, other rehabilitation staff reported Mr. Robinson was noncompliant, with refusal to get out of bed or perform exercises. At the initial interview, Mr. Robinson reported that he was retired from the Air Force. He also reported that he had actively participated in a health club, walking and exercising daily with his spouse. Additionally, he reported a hobby of woodworking. His home included a woodshop in which he built grandfather clocks, furniture, and other intricate pieces. His affect clearly brightened when discussing his woodworking. Mr. Robinson indicated that he wanted to return to his previous activity level of independence in activities of daily living and exercise at the health club, as well as woodworking. He had shortness of breath and fatigue throughout the interview and needed to return from sitting upright to supine after 15 minutes. At the conclusion of the interview, it was mutually agreed on that Mr. Robinson would assess a new Dremel that was recently acquired by the therapist and explain its various parts and functions.

The following day, Mr. Robinson sat on the side of the bed for 20 minutes in the morning and 30 minutes in the afternoon while enthusiastically reaching for various accessories of the Dremel and explaining their purposes. (Mr. Robinson continued to refuse the physical therapist's requests to get out of bed and exercise or to go to the gym for group exercise.)

On the second day, the occupational therapist brought wood and asked Mr. Robinson if he would like to make something. He replied, "No, but I would love to show you how to use the Dremel." The therapist then suggested that he get out of bed and into a wheelchair so they could go to the gym for the instruction. Mr. Robinson then donned his robe with minimum assistance, transferred to the chair with contact guard assistance, and went to the gym.

Mr. Robinson carefully scanned the environment of the gym, observing other patients and activities. In a quiet room adjacent to the gym, Mr. Robinson sat in the wheelchair while drawing designs on wood and demonstrating the use of the Dremel. When fatigued, he would have the therapist use the Dremel and then inspect her work. Mr. Robinson tolerated being out of bed in the wheelchair for 30 minutes in the morning and 30 minutes in the afternoon.

During these sessions, the therapist and Mr. Robinson discussed his heart attack that had led to the bypass procedure, and the fears and anxieties he had about resuming activity. In addition, before, during, and after each session, oxygen saturation levels were taken and recorded by Mr. Robinson following initial instruction on oximeter use. The therapist pointed out increased tolerance of activity as evidenced by gains in sitting tolerance, standing tolerance, and time out of bed.

The following morning, Mr. Robinson was dressed and ready to go to the gym for another Dremel lesson. (He still refused to participate in individual or group exercise.) This time the therapist asked Mr. Robinson to stand at the counter to do the demonstration and critique the therapist's use of the tool. Mr. Robinson tolerated standing for the lesson for 15 minutes, a 10-minute rest in his chair, and then another 15 minutes of standing. During the lesson, Mr. Robinson asked, "Did you hear it?" The therapist replied, "Hear what?" Mr. Robinson said, "Why, the sound of the wood talking to you." He pointed out that when the tool cut through various grains of wood, the sounds varied with the hardness of the wood. Mr. Robinson clearly loved his work with wood, was highly knowledgeable about woodworking, and easily engaged in this familiar and comfortable activity.

In the afternoon, Mr. Robinson stated that he would like to try some exercising in the gym. He did some lower and upper extremity exercises (without weights or resistance and no upper extremity movements over 90 degrees). The following morning Mr. Robinson participated in the full rehabilitation program and continued to be active and "in compliance" through discharge and outpatient rehabilitation.

Case contributed by Joanna Lipoma, MOT, OTR

Case 10-4

The New Resident

I worked with a 95-year-old woman who was admitted to our skilled nursing facility with hospice services. Hospice automatically makes one ineligible for therapy except in a few circumstances, so following this admission, she went without therapeutic intervention for several months. Before admission, she had lived in an assisted living facility. She needed minimal assistance for self-care and followed a self-designed and highly specific routine. She had significant visual impairments due to macular degeneration but still enjoyed choosing her own outfits, feeding herself, and propelling her wheelchair independently. She spent most of her time socializing with friends. Over the course of her time in the skilled nursing facility, her physical condition deteriorated so that she required maximal to total assistance for all self-care and a Hoyer lift for functional transfers. She was isolated in her room. Her family was finally able to advocate for a discharge from hospice. I was then asked to evaluate her.

Without hesitation, she was able to give a long, detailed list of the things she wanted to do; she had plenty of desire for mastery, but the social environment (staff) and physical environment were thwarting her, providing no "just-right" press or challenge. She wanted to feed herself, but she could not visually locate items on her plate. She wanted to participate in dressing, but no one asked her what she wanted to wear. She wanted to wash her face herself, but the staff kept trying to give her generic soap instead of the salon products that she had in her drawer. She wanted to spend time out of bed, but the wheelchair she had been given was not comfortable. Additionally, the environment imposed the staff's occupational role expectation that this woman was a hospice patient, was dying, and was not capable of autonomy. Their role was to care for her, and her role was to passively accept. She was particularly loquacious, a quality the staff did not value. For example, they knew how to do a bed bath and did not need her constant input or instruction. When the staff would not listen to her, she stopped participating in her own self-care. Not surprisingly, she reported experiencing depression and little desire for mastery.

After lengthy discussions with her to develop a shared vision, the bulk of the interventions I provided to my client involved educating the staff on the client's needs and desires and creating a supportive physical environment. The physical environmental interventions of finding a better-fitting wheelchair, new shoes with traction for self-propelling, and a visor to shield her eyes from bright lights were easy. Changing the staff's role expectations was harder but resulted in a greater chance for adaptation. I had to convince them that she was not a dying, dependent woman. She deserved their respect, and they could, in fact, learn from her about how to do their jobs (bed baths included). When she was given opportunities and learned that her desires were respected, she was able to adapt in many ways and increased her sense of relative mastery. She began to feed herself independently after developing a series of questions to ask the staff about where items were and instructing them to rearrange her plate for easier access. Even more impressively, she felt confident enough to voice a formal complaint when she felt she was being mistreated by a particular staff member, a feat she would not have attempted when I first met her. She was now able to seek her own justice.

Case contributed by Jennifer K. Whittaker, MSOT, OTR/L, CPH, CHES

By facilitating renewed desires for mastery, the resident was empowered to regain her autonomy in some very important ways, thus improving her performance skills and her quality of life. Although on the verge of giving up entirely, she had not fully internalized the external expectations of the facility staff. Thanks to the advocacy of her family and her occupational therapist, she was able to tap into 95 years of adaptive repertoire to continue generating adaptive responses to occupational challenges in her new environment at the skilled nursing facility. Simultaneously, the occupational therapist was able to shift portions of the physical, social, and cultural occupational environment that, if integrated and sustained, will better serve many more residents in the future.

A Deeper Dive

When you are ready for a challenge, consider one or both of the following activities to strengthen your ability to plan effective occupational therapy interventions:

1. Take the Therapeutic Ingredients worksheet and, instead of adding the theory, add a specific plan for how to implement each ingredient with a particular client (person, group, or population).

2. Use the Therapeutic Ingredients worksheet to guide your observation of good therapists at work. Note how they implement various therapeutic ingredients into practice from your viewpoint. Following the session, ask about the rationale behind each of their choices in the therapy session.

TAKE-AWAY MESSAGES

◊ Intervention is centered around enabling participation in a relevant, meaningful occupational role.

◊ The therapist learns about the desired occupational role from the client.

◊ The focus of intervention is on facilitating adaptive responses within valued occupational roles.

◊ The therapist acts as an agent of the occupational environment to provide just-right occupational challenges and facilitate adaptive responses.

◊ The client operates as the agent of internal change that taps into and enhances adaptive capacity.

References

Abreu, B. C. (2011). Accentuate the positive: Reflections on empathic interpersonal interactions (Eleanor Clarke Slagle lecture). *American Journal of Occupational Therapy, 65*, 623-634. https://doi.org/10.5014/ajot.2011.656002

Bachman, S. (2016). Evidence-based approach to treating lateral epicondylitis using the occupational adaptation model. *American Journal of Occupational Therapy, 70*, 7002360010. https://doi.org/10.5014/ajot.2016.016972

Christiansen, C. H. (1999). Defining lives: Occupation as identity: An essay on competence, coherence, and the creation of meaning, 1999 Eleanor Clarke Slagle lecture. *American Journal of Occupational Therapy, 53*, 547-558. https://doi.org/10.5014/ajot.53.6.547

Cole, M. B., & Tufano, R. (2008). Occupational Adaptation. In M. B. Cole & R. Tufano (Eds.), *Applied theories in occupational therapy: A practical approach* (2nd ed., pp. 107-115). SLACK Incorporated.

George-Paschal, L., & Bowen, M. R. (2019). Outcomes of a mentoring program based on occupational adaptation for participants in a juvenile drug court program. *Occupational Therapy in Mental Health, 35*(3), 262-286. https://doi.org/10.1080/0164212X.2019.1601605

Gillen, G. (2013). A fork in the road: An occupational hazard? (Eleanor Clarke Slagle lecture). *American Journal of Occupational Therapy, 67*(6), 641-652. https://doi.org/10.5014/ajot.2013.676002

Giles, G. M. (2018). Neurocognitive rehabilitation: Skills or strategies? *The American Journal of Occupational Therapy, 72*(6), 7206150010p1-7206150010p16.

Grejo, L. C. (2017). Occupational adaptation. In J. Hinojosa, P. Kramer, & C. B. Royeen (Eds.), *Perspectives on human occupation: Theories underlying practice* (2nd ed., pp. 287-311). F. A. Davis.

Law, M. (2002). Participation in the occupations of everyday life. *The American Journal of Occupational Therapy, 56*(6), 640-649.

Mitcham, M. D. (2014). Education as engine (Eleanor Clarke Slagle lecture). *American Journal of Occupational Therapy, 68*, 636-648. https://doi.org/10.5014/ajot.2014.686001

Schultz, S. (2014). Theory of occupational adaptation. In H. S. Willard & B. A. B. Schell (Eds.), *Willard & Spackman's occupational therapy* (12th ed., pp. 527-540). Wolters Kluwer Health/Lippincott Williams & Wilkins.

Stelter, L. D., & Evetts, C. L. (2020). Effect of an occupation-based program for women with intellectual and developmental disabilities who are incarcerated. *Annals of International Occupational Therapy, 3*(4), 175-184. https://doi.org/10.3928/24761222-20190910-01

Stelter, L., & Whisner, S. M. (2007). Building responsibility for self through meaningful roles: Occupational adaptation theory applied in forensic psychiatry. *Occupational Therapy in Mental Health, 23*(1), 69-84.

A DEEPER DIVE WORKSHEET

Therapeutic Ingredients

For each of the recommended therapeutic ingredients, write a statement that links the intervention strategy to the theory of occupational adaptation and answers the following question: "Why is this important?"

THERAPEUTIC INGREDIENT	WHY? (LINK TO THEORY)
Intentionally provide opportunities to select, plan, and execute meaningful activity and evaluate task performance	
Intentionally provide opportunities to create tangible products or intangible but recognizable outcomes	
Intentionally provide opportunities to engage in graded, just-right occupational challenges	
Intentionally provide opportunities to receive direct or indirect verbal or physical assistance only as necessary	
Intentionally provide opportunities to receive objective, nonjudgmental feedback	
Intentionally provide opportunities to participate in novel tasks or contexts	
Intentionally provide opportunities to engage in a positive social environment	
Intentionally provide opportunities to experience self in an occupational role that is personally satisfying	

Evetts, C. L., & Baxter, M. F. (2024). *Cases and Concepts in Occupational Adaptation: Translating Theory into Action*. SLACK Incorporated.

CHAPTER **11**

Documentation and Dissemination, Interprofessional and Intraprofessional Communication

How Do You Describe Occupational Adaptation to Others?

> *One of the toughest challenges in occupational therapy is to talk explicitly about what seems so evident to us because we assume it's evident to everyone else.*
> —Maralynne D. Mitcham (2014, p. 643)

Documentation: Communicating With the Team and Reimbursers

Imagine that you just finished a delightfully meaningful therapy session; the goals your client worked so hard to achieve culminated in a successful outcome, and you head toward the charting room feeling like something great has been accomplished. Now comes a new challenge—capturing the magic in writing. Effectively using the written language to convey the medical necessity and skilled components of an intervention is critical to ensure reimbursement, communicate with team members about a client's status, and justify the need for occupational therapy.

In settings such as hospitals, nursing homes, and rehabilitation centers, occupational therapists must establish that their services are medically necessary to be covered by insurance. Insurers may stipulate that therapy be justified by a reasonable expectation that improvement will be made and that therapeutic intervention is required to prevent further debility. Using an occupational adaptation approach helps therapists capture progress in a uniquely nuanced manner,

Evetts, C. L., & Baxter, M. F. *Cases and Concepts in Occupational Adaptation: Translating Theory into Action* (pp. 99-104).
DOI: 10.4324/9781003522850-11

which is critically important in instances in which an occupational therapist's documentation contributes to decisions, such as the length of therapy service allotment. Regardless of the setting, occupational therapists use documentation to articulate the need for the profession's specific skill set. In other words, although a therapist may know what they are doing with a client, the inability to clearly articulate the need for skilled services may lead to costly reimbursement challenges.

On another note, occupational therapists use documentation to communicate with team members. Evaluations, daily notes, and progress notes articulate the plan of care, identify areas of strength and weakness, and describe the progress toward goals. Any of these functions might facilitate continuity of care among team members. A patient's nurse may review occupational therapy documentation on the individual's functional transfers before assisting the patient to bed. The patient's physician may review occupational therapy notes to monitor progress in self-care. There is another benefit to clear communication in this realm; consider the instances when a member of the patient's care team is confused about why the patient seemed to be leisurely knitting during occupational therapy time. Skillful occupational therapy notes offer the opportunity to communicate the intentionality and theoretical underpinnings of occupation-based services. Watching a therapist engage a client in meaningful occupations may lack context, particularly to anyone unfamiliar with the profession or the occupational adaptation framework. Documentation is the place to clarify the why, how, and so-what of it all.

To the final point, clear documentation bolsters the profession of occupational therapy. To an outsider who is not privy to the multifaceted plans of an occupational therapist, it may appear that they are doing the same job as a nursing technician when engaging a client in a showering activity or a recreation therapist when the client is completing crafts. Documentation is one of the fundamental ways occupational therapists communicate the unique benefits of their professional skill set. Using occupation-based theories and language only adds to the authenticity of occupational therapy practice.

Repeated Measures of Baseline Skills

We can observe adaptive behavior and infer that adaptation has occurred, but how is that documented in objective ways that convince others that the intervention is working? Recall that, contrary to treatment approaches that assume if a client gains skills they will become adaptive, an occupational adaptation approach proposes that when a client becomes more adaptive, they will demonstrate skilled performance. Therefore, measure skills at baseline, but focus treatment on occupational challenges that tap into desire and press for mastery. Then, reassess skill to document change.

Change in Attitude, Affect, Approach, and Adaptation

The section heading suggests four strategies an occupational therapist can use to detect a change outside the realm of performance: alteration in attitude, affect, approach, and adaptation. Each of these areas offers insight into the workings of the internal adaptation process and may be helpful in describing to others what you mean by "adaptation." Because the ultimate goal is to foster an adaptive response, occupational therapists applying this theory should monitor these responses as indicators of meaningful change. In other words, although an individual's performance may technically remain static between two sessions, a change in attitude or affect could signify a shift in the inner workings of the adaptation process. For example, picture a client who presents to therapy services with a pessimistic, fearful, or critical attitude and a sour or flat affect. Occupational adaptation tells us that a person's desire for mastery is critical to the press for mastery and occupational response; furthermore, adaptive response evaluation is an internal process influenced by the individual's state of mind. Until the therapist helps the individual tap into the ever-present desire for mastery, the client will be hard-pressed to make meaningful gains in therapy. As the desire for mastery is identified, goals established, and rapport built, the therapist may witness the client's attitude shift toward optimism, confidence, or curiosity with a brighter or more animated affect. Here, the adaptation process is at work.

Approach and adaptation are two additional areas worthy of documentation. You might recall that during adaptive response evaluation, a person gauges their performance through the lens of relative mastery (i.e., how efficient, effective, and satisfactory the performance was). A change in approach is an external indicator of the adaptive response generation process functioning. Performance occurred, the person evaluated that their performance was unsatisfactory in some way, and as a result of that assessment, the person changed their tactics. An observant therapist will take note of the adaptive modes the client uses (existing, modified, or new) and the pattern of adaptive response behaviors (stable, mobile, or blended), all of which offer insight into the adaptation process. Furthermore, paying thoughtful attention to the adaptation process in your documentation substantiates skillful application of occupational therapy services. Next, let us consider ways to document that adaptation has truly occurred.

Initiation of Adaptive Responses in Novel Situations

One way to document that the adaptation process is at work is to offer novel challenges during therapy sessions. Although an adaptive strategy may be masterfully applied in a task familiar to the individual, changing an element of the occupation (perhaps through the location, the materials, or the amount of cuing) can drastically alter the experience. The ability to initiate adaptive strategies for novel challenges is a more powerful indication of change than task mastery alone.

As an example, picture a client, Marcel, who presented to occupational therapy in an acute care hospital. Marcel and his care team were concerned about his ability to dress himself while following spinal precautions (i.e., no bending, lifting, or twisting). Marcel's morning occupational therapy session focused on education about spinal precautions and an introduction to adaptive equipment. He demonstrated understanding of how to use a reacher to don a pair of pants from sitting on the edge of his hospital bed. Marcel's therapist noted that he demonstrated mastery over a task using hospital pants but planned to offer novel challenges to test Marcel's ability to initiate the use of adaptive tools in a different occupational context. This would indicate whether Marcel had learned to complete a specific task (i.e., donning hospital pants with a reacher) or whether adaptive equipment use represented a new or modified adaptive response mode.

In the afternoon session, the therapist acted as an agent of the environment to facilitate the following novel challenges:

- Used Marcel's street clothes for dressing instead of loose hospital scrubs
- Integrated item retrieval because his clothes were on a low shelf across the room
- Challenged Marcel to change into his own clothing in preparation for discharge home using any strategy that seemed effective but remained safe

Up to this point, Marcel had only demonstrated the ability to don a pair of hospital pants with the reacher. However, when presented with novel tasks, he seamlessly applied use of the adaptive tool to gather clothing from a shelf too low to comfortably reach, to doff his hospital pants and socks, and to thread his feet through his jeans. Marcel demonstrated integration of an adaptive response by applying compensatory strategies across novel challenges in an activity of daily living environment. Furthermore, as the session progressed and Marcel experienced repeated success with his newfound tool, he reflected out loud that he could likely use the reacher for other tasks too—"I bet this could help me reach the laundry or the dog bowl on the floor." Marcel's statements are further indications that his adaptive capacity is expanding beyond the occupational challenges faced in the hospital to serve him well when he returns home.

In summary, document skills, subtle changes that point to an internal adaptation process occurring, and spontaneous initiation of adaptive strategies in novel situations. Long-term goals reflect meaningful occupational roles. Short-term goals relate to elements within the occupational adaptation process, needed changes within the adaptive response mechanism, and shifts in adaptation energy, modes, behaviors, and/or gestalt.

Dissemination: Explaining the Occupational Adaptation Approach

Now that you have walked through the occupational adaptation process for yourself in the Try It On exercises, you are ready to focus on how to introduce and explain the process to others. We have had successful outcomes and positive feedback with the following approaches in both academic and clinical settings. Our experience as clinicians and educators has taught us the importance of being able to articulate what we are doing that makes us different from others. As you have experienced for yourself in this book, practicing from this framework is distinctively different than practicing from other frequently used perspectives in the clinical arena. Let us discuss the different case scenarios that you might experience and the strategy of "telling it like it is" to various audiences. We have chosen four key components of occupational adaptation to characterize these discussions: (a) holistic model for practice, (b) the client is the agent of change, (c) every client has desire for mastery, and (d) the client is involved in evaluation. In the following sections, we demonstrate how we use these four pillars to shape clear, relevant conversations with physicians, the clinical community, and other occupational therapists.

The Physician

We all know that the physician's time is limited. We need to address issues quickly and concisely, "get in and get out," as we tell our occupational therapy interns. Whether you are selling occupational therapy for an initial consult or rationalizing your approach to treatment, the major assumptions of occupational adaptation are the ticket in this situation. They have been threaded throughout the guide and re-emphasized here.

Holistic

Although there are many disciplines using the term *holistic*, it is important that you take a few moments to explain how your approach addresses the whole person (i.e., body structures and functions, performance skills, and performance patterns). It has been our experience that in a physical dysfunction setting, physicians have been surprised that occupational therapy addresses more than motor components. This is why in treatment team meetings, the occupational therapist practicing from an occupational adaptation perspective reports on patients' processing skills and communication and interaction responses while engaged in activities of daily living or other occupational tasks. Likewise, in psychiatric settings, physicians have been enlightened that occupational therapy is incorporating sensory, motor, and cognitive functions when seeing patients. This explains why the occupational therapist practicing from an occupational adaptation theoretical perspective is not limiting services to paper-and-pencil counseling sessions but including other meaningful activities to remediate functional deficits in moving and thinking.

The Client Is the Agent of Change

Remember that the typical physician population comes from the traditional medical model. They are used to doing procedures to their clients and/or prescribing drugs that the patient takes to facilitate an internal chemical change. Historically, a patient under a physician's care does not question the recommended treatment and/or medicine being prescribed. Therefore, it is essential that you describe how your approach focuses on empowering the client to be the agent of change while you the occupational therapist are active in "setting the stage" by designing the environment for client adaptation to occur. It is oftentimes at this point that the physician understands patient reports of doing "strange" activities in occupational therapy sessions, such as flower arranging, fishing with hip wader boots, and so on, all of which are performed with "real" materials. We find that physicians often ask, "How did you know how to do that? Do you fish in the swamps?" This is the perfect opening to boast about our patients' involvement in designing their own occupational therapy treatment challenges. Not to mention, this involvement requires the patient to engage a great deal of cognitive effort to teach the occupational therapist about swamp fishing!

Every Client Has a Desire for Mastery

Briefly describe how you believe that every client (use their client as an example) has a desire to master something. We have found that stating our "trick of the trade" is the client's primary occupational role, and we go from there. We often reiterate at this point that those clients, being agents and directors of their own occupational therapy challenges, get "fired up" to master the activities that the occupational therapist provides. Isn't it true that when our patients are engaged in activities they want to master, they give their best effort?

The Client Is Involved With the Evaluation Process

Physicians need to know that the "secret of your success" is that the patient and occupational therapist collaboratively and dynamically evaluate the patient's response to the challenges being addressed in occupational therapy. The treatment process from initial assessment through discharge is formulated and altered by the clients' evaluation of whether or not they feel they are efficient, effective, and satisfied with their progress and performance.

The Clinical Community

This category of individuals was hard to name because we find ourselves describing our approach to clinicians of other disciplines on the team, as well as other occupational therapists. Therefore, we approach this category encompassing all clinicians on the team. In our experience, the inquiries we receive about our approach to occupational therapy treatment are based on a treatment session they observe or ones in which they are directly involved (such as cotreatment sessions or team teaching) and/or feedback they hear from others. Using the "client in question" is the way to go. Use the specific case/class/client as the base for your description. We usually describe our approach using the general occupational adaptation assumptions and then go directly to the particular client and their primary occupational role. A description of the initiated treatment program then follows naturally. This is an excellent opportunity to help others understand the meaning behind what is being used to reach occupational therapy goals. We also explain what activities the occupational therapist is using as readiness and what challenges the client is engaged in that are occupational activities for that individual. This usually ends up with a discussion of why our clients do not all do the same things, even if they have a similar diagnosis and/or primary physician.

Often in treatment team meetings, we have had the experience of being consulted to offer suggestions for how to deal with a "difficult" client or one who is "unmotivated" for therapy. Our usual response is the following: "Did you ask the client what they want to do?" This is an automatic response from us because of the inherent assumption in occupational adaptation that the person has a desire to master something. Finding this something is what makes treatment so dynamic and individualistic. Telling it like it is involves educating others about the process and approach to treatment but also educating them on how to use the occupational adaptation approach to involve the client. It is not a novel concept to include the client in the evaluative process, but it is often overlooked and underemphasized. So, next time a fellow team member is brainstorming about what to do next with an "unmotivated" or "uncooperative" client, try asking what it is the client desires to do and whether that is being threaded into the therapeutic process. Part of our reward as occupational therapists practicing the occupational adaptation theory has been not only being a part of the relative mastery that our patients experience but also witnessing the relative mastery other team members experience when they can focus on their patients' primary occupational role, use it in treatment, and reap the rewards for their efforts!

The Occupational Therapist

This final section addresses the "inquiring mind" of the occupational therapist population. Often, occupational therapists have heard general information about occupational adaptation and know the basics of the framework. They often have case scenarios of their own that map out some of the cases presented or documented in publications. Their comments generally range from "This sounds like what I do" to "Isn't this what occupational therapy is all about?" It is at this point that these questions should be answered in-depth with the components of the occupational adaptation framework. Yes, it does require an element of time. Can you imagine if we attempted to engage you in the adaptive response subprocesses in one chapter in this book? Keep in mind that sufficiently answering questions from the inquisitive occupational therapist takes time. How long does it take? In the following sections, we attempt to separate and give suggestions for the common avenues that we have used.

The In-Service

Most occupational therapy departments have times set aside for staff in-services. This may be during a weekly staff meeting or a designated in-service time. Typically, the allotted time is about 1 hour, maybe less. This is not a tremendous amount of time to delve into some of the most complex aspects, such as the adaptive response subprocesses. Keep it simple; explain the major assumptions of occupational adaptation with emphasis on its uniqueness. Use a handout and/or slides of the visual model to identify the person, occupational environment, and interaction of these as challenges occur. We have found that providing a case example and then plugging that person into the schematic for explanation is beneficial. Do not be surprised if you get an invitation from the group to come back to explain further.

The Short Course or Workshop

The short course or workshop provides more time to really get into the occupational adaptation process. Initial time should be set aside to lay the foundation for the occupational adaptation framework. This includes history, assumptions, and unique characteristics of the theory. Next, describe the person and the occupational environment with specifics of the assumptions and components. We always have participants complete a short exercise illustrating these foundational concepts on themselves. The following time should be spent according to the people present in your short course or workshop. There are two methods to do this, each having their own strengths.

If you get the feeling that your group participants are game for a challenge and can wait awhile for a description of the role of the occupational therapist, then address the person first. This next chunk of time needs to be devoted to the three adaptive response subprocesses (i.e., generation, evaluation, and integration). This is our favorite part because we believe the unique flavor of this theory really comes alive when you begin to explore these. Have your participants engage in applying these concepts through short group activities, discussions, and/or paper description. We have personal examples before applying the theory to a patient. Finish with the occupational environment and its role in the occupational adaptation process.

The second way to delve into the occupational adaptation process (after explaining the general assumptions and description of the person and occupational environment) is to begin with the occupational environment. Why? We advocate beginning with the occupational environment when the group participants are pressing for "how" and "what role does the occupational therapist play." It is similar to the first method; however, you are beginning with the occupational environment and then following with the person and adaptive processes. Again, the method you use will depend on the group attending. Either way, it is always wise to finish your short course or workshop with time to explore a case and answer questions to sum up the experience.

The Institute or All-Day Workshop

An all-day workshop allows more time to illustrate the flow of the occupational adaptation process. We suggest group activities to facilitate understanding of the main occupational adaptation framework. Having an all-day workshop also gives the participants time to use the framework personally and professionally. Participation from the audience for examples of the occupational adaptation process "at work" in patient care is typically very contagious. Do not forget to allot time to describe the research being developed and documented with occupational adaptation. This book may help with references. Do not be afraid to write up some of your patient cases and use them as scenarios for discussion. It can be a great learning experience for you and the group participants. Consult the cases in this book for examples of how you might develop your application of occupational adaptation into case studies for discussion.

Reference

Mitcham, M. D. (2014). Education as engine (Eleanor Clarke Slagle lecture). *American Journal of Occupational Therapy, 68,* 636-648. https://doi.org/10.5014/ajot.2014.686001

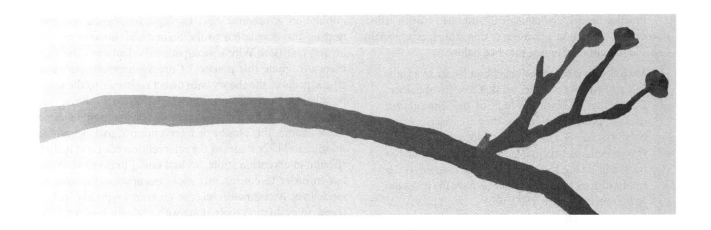

Occupational Adaptation Practice Models

*We might benefit as a profession if we were
more explicit about how we help people engage ...*
—Virginia Stoffel (2015, p. 3)

What Are Practice Models?

Practice models grounded in theory are developed to guide why, when, and how to provide intervention to a particular population; this leads to best practice. When a practice is carried out in an organized and systematic fashion, it is easier to conduct outcome studies that reveal the value of the practice. As Law (2002) points out, "The use of qualitative methods and more complex quantitative methods will enable researchers to disentangle the complex relationship among person, environment, and participation in occupations" (p. 645). When intake and outcome measures reflect individual client data, case studies can be developed. Single-subject design studies can be formed, and then over time, multiple cases can be compared. Cohort or population studies are possible when data are aggregated. When data represent deidentified information related to referrals, attendance, average length of intervention, rates of reinjury, or rate of change in comorbid conditions, program evaluation studies are possible. Documenting outcomes that show progress influences best practice when these reports are disseminated in our professional literature and presented at professional conferences.

Evetts, C. L., & Baxter, M. F. *Cases and Concepts in Occupational Adaptation:
Translating Theory into Action* (pp. 105-106).
DOI: 10.4324/9781003522850-12

Practice models are valuable to stimulate critical reflection on our evaluation and intervention strategies, especially to avoid the pitfall of falling into bad habits.

> My reflections led to the belief that we are in a rut, a valuable rut, but a rut for all that. We are not alone. Every other profession is in a rut, too. The ruts are made of professional habits. They are well worn and comfortable … For long-established professions this is, perhaps, acceptable but, for one as young as ours, still trying to explore its potential, the rut is inhibiting our becoming what we have the potential to become. (Wilcock, 1999, p. 7)

For decades an enduring conversation within occupational therapy has been the importance of embracing occupation as the core of the profession and the incorporation of occupation-based interventions in practice. The practice models that follow offer examples of practice that align with occupational adaptation principles, applying occupation-based and client-centered strategies to bring about meaningful change.

Upcoming Chapters

Each practice model presented in Chapters 12 and 13 follows the same basic structure. A rationale provides the fundamental reason for establishing the practice model. It describes the need for intervention with the particular population. A premise states the logic supporting and connecting the population to the theory and answers the following question: Why is occupational adaptation the right theory to guide this practice? Core assumptions state specific aspects of the theory with direct relevance to the target population. Next, effects of dysadaptation establish the consequences of not providing services, consultation, or direct intervention. The phases of intervention signal beginning, middle, and later stages of the intervention plan and include specific intervention strategies that ought to occur throughout in order to consistently apply occupational adaptation guidelines. Assessment/outcome measures typically include standard evaluation tools along with evaluation of issues related to adaptive capacity and relative mastery. Finally, the overall goal is reiterated. Following some practice models, a case is provided to illustrate how a client interaction followed the plan.

References

Law, M. C. (2002). Participation in the occupations of everyday life. *American Journal of Occupational Therapy, 56*(6), 640-649. https://doi.org/10.5014/ajot.56.6.640

Stoffel, V. (2015). Engagement, exploration, empowerment. *The American Journal of Occupational Therapy, 69*(6), 6906140010p1-6906140010p8.

Wilcock, A. A. (1999). Reflections on doing, being, and becoming. *Australian Occupational Therapy Journal, 46,* 1-11.

Practice Models Highlighting Occupational Adaptation Across the Life Span

Engagement in occupation implies
being involved, making choices, and taking risks.
Occupational performance is an experience
rather than an observed phenomenon—
a feature of all humans, regardless of age, gender, or disability.
—Mary C. Law (2007)

Occupational adaptation principles can be applied to clients in any stage of life. We present four practice models that exemplify practice with various age groups, including children, adolescents, adults, and older adults. As you read, consider how the models might be adapted to your practice.

Evetts, C. L., & Baxter, M. F. *Cases and Concepts in Occupational Adaptation:*
Translating Theory into Action (pp. 107-117).
DOI: 10.4324/9781003522850-13

Practice Model 12-1: Occupational Adaptation Approach to Pediatric Feeding Disorders in Intensive Outpatient Therapy

Submitted by Jessica Johnson, OTR, MOT

Rationale

Feeding disorders are prevalent in up to 80% of children with complex medical issues and are highly heterogeneous (Edwards et al., 2015, 2016; Fishbein et al., 2016). It is estimated that 4 in 100,000 children require enteral nutrition (i.e., the practice of delivering nutrition through a tube to the stomach; Edwards et al., 2016), which is necessary for children who are unwilling or are unable to meet their nutritional needs. A multidisciplinary approach to treatment is indicated as best practice for this population to address the multidimensional nature of feeding difficulties (Edwards et al., 2016; Fishbein et al., 2016; Sharp et al., 2017). The development of eating skills is complex and, for typically developing children, covers up to a 3-year process (Rudolph & Link, 2002). Children who receive tube feedings lack both skill and experience to be successful oral feeders for several reasons. Addressing the multidimensional skill limitations while also providing holistic care is challenging, particularly in a cost-containment environment, such as an outpatient setting, where the number of visits for therapeutic intervention is dictated by payer sources.

Premise

- The occupational adaptation framework allows occupational therapists to consider the depth and complexity of demands placed on each person in the child–caregiver dyad. Thus, therapists can better define their role within a multidisciplinary team to facilitate the dyad's adaptive process within mealtime challenges.
- Successful mealtimes are not solely defined by the volume of oral intake. This practice model is intended to guide the clinician in their assessment of the press for mastery between the person and environmental factors and create interventions to facilitate successful occupational engagement in family and social mealtimes.

- Considering the adaptive gestalt of the dyad, as opposed to solely the observable behavior, can aid the clinician in problem setting to best support the client's successful occupational engagement.
- Family participation is critical in the program's success because the primary caregiver is a member of the dyad and the collective family unit that provides an environmental press for mastery. The occupational therapist will help the family set realistic, attainable goals that will best meet the expectations of the individual in the context of the family. The 5-week program lays the foundation for the family to help their child engage successfully in mealtimes in their natural environment upon discharge.

Core Assumptions

- The child and their caregiver are viewed as each being made up of the following holistic person systems: performance patterns, performance skills (motor, process, and interaction), and shared personal context. All elements are present and active in the dyad with every feeding response.
- The dyad intends to produce a response to a mealtime challenge that will be adaptive, and therefore, will lead to mastery.
- Relative mastery is the extent to which the child–caregiver dyad experiences the feeding response as efficient (use of time and energy), effective (production of the desired result), and satisfying to self and society (i.e., it is pleasing not only to the self but also to the relevant others as agents of the occupational environment).
- When confronted with a mealtime challenge that is beyond the dyad's current capabilities, hyperstable engagement in pre-existing strategies is normative when used as a temporary balance-restoring strategy.
- The dyad's state of occupational functioning is changed as a result of an occupational event. One of three states of occupational functioning is reinforced as a result: occupational adaptation, homeostasis, or occupational dysadaptation.

Effects of Occupational Dysadaptation

The gastrostomy tube serves as a medical intervention to allow these children to grow without the need for them to complete the preoral, oral, pharyngeal, or esophageal phases of normal feeding. Children who are tube fed have a history of dysadaptive eating patterns. Dysadaptation in feeding can result in food refusals, failure to thrive, oral aversions, recurrent pneumonia, chronic lung disease, or recurrent emesis (Rudolph & Link, 2002), which are common reasons for referral to outpatient feeding programs.

When a child experiences fear, pain, or discomfort at any phase of feeding, a child's adaptive response is negatively reinforced. Dependent on the environmental feedback, these adaptive response modes can be adaptive or dysadaptive. For example, if a child vomits with ingestion of a particular nutritional source, they may demonstrate an existing adaptive response mode and a hyperstable behavior where they stop eating. This is an adaptive behavior because it is preventing further discomfort for the child, and they have experienced relative mastery by increasing their comfort level and ending the meal for them to recover. However, this hyperstable adaptive response becomes dysadaptive if the child continues to generate this response each time they are presented with food items because they will not receive proper nutrition to grow.

Intervention Phases and Strategies

The role of the occupational therapist is that of a facilitator. As a facilitator, the occupational therapist designs, alters, and modifies the occupational environment and guides the child and caregiver as they participate in relevant occupational challenges. The occupational therapist's physical presence should be faded out of the immediate occupational environment by the start of the fifth week of programming to empower the family for discharge.

Overview of Occupational Therapy Processes
Initial Assessment

- Team evaluation includes the parents/caregivers, child, occupational therapist, speech-language pathologist, dietician, and psychologist. The goal of this evaluation is to determine program placement and a comprehensive understanding of feeding performance.
- Intake paperwork includes the following: chart review of prior records, demographics, history, food diary, current schedule, family concerns, sensory checklist, caregiver questionnaires, and description of refusal/maladaptive mealtime behaviors.

- Day of assessment/intake includes the following:
  - Arena assessment with role delineation, consistent with a multidisciplinary approach. Occupational therapy's role in assessment is to gather data regarding the child's sensorimotor, cognitive, and psychosocial functioning, whether through direct observation, parent interview, or coordination of care with other disciplines, and assess the occupational environment.
  - Formal developmental assessment is typically gathered from chart review or will be conducted within the first session of the treatment program, if necessary.
  - Detailed feeding history from birth is obtained and shared with all team members.
  - Mealtime observation with child and primary feeder, further parent interview, and additional clinical observations are conducted.
- Problem setting: Therapist guides the client through activity analysis of relevant mealtime tasks and sets SMART (specific, measurable, achievable, relevant, and time-bound) goals that include the language of relative mastery.

Occupational Therapy Interventions

- Occupational therapy is scheduled before speech-feeding therapy session to prepare the child for feeding activities.
- Occupational readiness: Foundational body structure and body function readiness with particular attention paid to oral sensory, oral and fine motor skills, postural control, and positioning.
- Occupational challenges are graded to meet the child where they are developmentally. Occupational environmental modifications and assistive devices can be used to facilitate a just-right challenge. Cultural and personal relevance is essential when setting up the occupational challenge and environment.

Overview of Intervention Methods

There are a variety of treatment methods that can be used due to the heterogeneity of this population (Edwards et al., 2016; Sharp et al., 2010, 2017). Best practices include behavioral intervention, sensorimotor skill building, activities of daily living training, environmental/task modifications, motor learning, and caregiver education.

Suggested Phases of Intervention

The time frames for the following phases are approximate and may vary:

- Phase I: The first 2 weeks of treatment are focused on occupational readiness with treatment activities designed by the therapist but relevant to the client's roles, routines, and preferences. The therapist facilitates foundational skill building, exploration, and education as appropriate for the dyad.
- Phase II: Involvement of the caregiver becomes the predominant focus of the next 2 weeks of treatment. Caregiver-selected food items, with guidance from the therapy team for safety, are encouraged, and child and caregiver-directed play and other mealtime activities are facilitated by the therapist. Home programming is encouraged during these 2 weeks to facilitate generalization of skills to the family's home environment.
- Phase III: The focus on week 5 interventions is discharge planning. The therapist begins to fade their presence within the occupational environment to further facilitate generalization of skills to the family's home environment. Home programming and reassessment are included in Phase III.

Outcome Measures

Typical outcome measures may include any of the following:

- Children's Eating and Behavior Inventory
- Mealtime Behavior Questionnaire
- Pediatric Evaluation of Disability Inventory
- Roll Evaluation of Activities of Life
- Hawaii Early Learning Profile Checklist
- Objective measurements of oral intake volume
- Food diaries

These outcome measures reflect skill acquisition, not relative mastery, and may not reflect qualitative changes in tolerance of mealtime or adaptive responses.

Occupational Adaptation Outcome Measures

Activity analysis can be an effective tool to guide the client through problem setting so that they may define efficiency, effectiveness, and satisfaction to self and others (Pasek & Schkade, 1996). Elements of relative mastery, as defined by the child–caregiver dyad, can then be embedded into the wording of long-term and short-term therapy goals to ensure relevance for client-centered practice. Lastly, goal attainment scaling can be completed by the caregiver upon reassessment

to measure progress toward relative mastery. Improvements in efficiency and effectiveness of mealtime reflect the child–caregiver dyad's synchronicity, and therefore, could be measured together. Cue-based algorithms, pain scales, and verbal reports from children are important measures of the child's satisfaction, as well as parent perception as the relevant other in the dyad. The therapist could also complete a satisfaction rating as relevant personnel in the dyad's occupational environment, which could be useful in considerations for discharge planning.

Overall Goal

The goal of this approach is to facilitate relative mastery of meaningful, mealtime occupations expected of the dyad to increase participation in the co-occupation of feeding. The goal is not to "fix" the child but rather to facilitate the child and caregiver's ability to adapt to new feeding challenges through relevant and satisfactory engagement in mealtime occupations that will improve the quality and participation of the child in family mealtimes in the home environment.

Practice Model 12-2: Preferred Interest Groups for Elementary School Students

Submitted by Christene Maas, PhD, MA, OTR

Rationale

The prevalence of children with autism spectrum disorder (ASD) is 1 in 36 individuals (Centers for Disease Control and Prevention [CDC], 2023b). As these children age, there continues to be a need for services to support them around the core deficit of social participation and relationships. A National Autism Indicators Report about the transition into young adulthood indicated that many individuals with ASD struggle with transition after high school to employment, independent living, and friendships (Roux et al., 2015). In social and community participation, individuals with ASD may have emerging social skills to function in the community yet continue to have difficulty making friends easily and are therefore at risk for experiencing greater loneliness, less satisfaction with their friendships than typical peers, and social isolation (Bauminger & Kasari, 2000; Roux et al., 2015). Conversely, research indicates an increase in social behavior during participation in preferred interests for both young children and high school–aged children (Dunst et al., 2012; Koegel et al., 2013; Koenig & Williams, 2017).

Schultz and Schkade (1992) asserted that for behaviors to become part of their adaptive response pattern, the internal adaptive process must be in a socially relevant activity. Participation in a group can facilitate the internal adaptive process by providing opportunities for relative mastery with the environmental press from a peer group (Pasek & Schkade, 1996; Schultz & Schkade, 1992). An occupational adaptation practice model using preferred interests or strength-based approaches within a group setting may help children with ASD to build adaptive response repertoires they can generalize to their next group activity.

Premise

Intervention within a school or community setting for children with ASD provides a naturalistic context that demands mastery to generalize the adaptive response process.

- The use of groups with children and adolescents supports the internal occupational adaptation process by presenting an occupational role in the occupational environment with specific physical, social, and cultural demands.
- Using preferred interests as a strength-based approach for individuals with ASD influences desire for mastery and a meaningful press for mastery.
- Occupational therapists are in a unique position to address aspects of the adaptation gestalt, such as sensory processing issues and emotional regulation, that, when out of balance, may affect social participation within the group context.

Core Assumptions

- The occupational environment is part of the external expectation and feedback in occupational adaptation theory, which begins with a demand for mastery from the environment. The occupational environment consists of physical, social, and cultural contexts. Individuals with ASD may have difficulties using context to construct meaning (Vermeulen, 2015).
- Demands to perform happen as part of the person's occupational roles and context in which they occur, also known as the *person-occupational environment interactions* (Schultz, 2014).
- Individuals generate adaptive responses when presented with a desired occupational challenge.
- The occupational challenge of social participation can be addressed by using a preferred interest to increase the desire for mastery for children with ASD.

Effects of Occupational Dysadaptation

One of the primary occupational challenges for individuals with ASD is social participation within a group. In a socially situated occupational challenge, students with ASD may have difficulty with social participation that requires joint attention, social referencing, flexibility, and perspective taking within interactions. One's adaptation gestalt can affect social participation when, for example, sensory functions are unmodulated or interaction skills do not meet external expectations. In addition, individuals with ASD may have "context blindness," which is the lack of using contextual sensitivity to construct meaning (Vermeulen, 2015). Therefore, children with ASD can have deficits with the social inferencing and self-regulation needed when talking with peers, which eventually affects making and maintaining friendships. The result for those with ASD can ultimately be loneliness and lack of satisfaction with friendships.

Intervention Phases and Strategies

Occupational Readiness

To start the group session, the occupational therapist will incorporate a self-regulation activity lasting for 60 seconds from https://calmclassroom.com/ to address the sensorimotor and psychosocial gestalt of the students before starting the activity (Benson & Wilcher, 2000; Calm Classroom, 2016). Clear concise directions with a visual schedule of the group are placed at the front, along with visual supports for activity goals. This utilizes strengths of individuals with ASD as visual learners, as well as addresses the adaptation gestalt.

Intervention During Groups

The use of strategies from the Zones of Regulation program and Social Thinking curriculum during the group supports self-regulation, social cognition or social thinking strategies, and perspective taking. These methods aid in the evaluating and integrating of new adaptive responses into the adaptive repertoire. Reflection of observations from the last session should be done to facilitate integrating new adaptive responses into the adaptive repertoire. Based on Schkade and Schultz (2003), the occupational therapist is not making suggestions but rather observations of positive or negative interactions and using therapeutic use of self. Specific group activities using preferred interests with the "just-right" occupational challenge can be used to address the following: joint attention, sharing of materials, flexibility, and working together in dyads initially to complete a project. A "toolbox" notebook for strategies should be used, including pictures from prior sessions for supporting episodic memory and visual strategies from previous sessions that can generalize to support adaptive response integration.

Phases of Typical Intervention

- An 8-week group of homogenous peers with a common interest is formed. For example, peers may form a group for building LEGOs (The Lego Group), learning about dinosaurs, playing ping-pong, or baking cookies. The importance is that the actual activity is not prescribed but rather is chosen by each member of the group.
- Homogenous group: The first step includes only children with ASD. As an after-school or community group, the selected activity should be repeated in this process as often as the individual with ASD chooses to participate.
- If generalization is not occurring within the homogenous group, the occupational therapist can evaluate to assess whether additional individual intervention is needed to promote occupational readiness.
- Heterogeneous group: After completion of the homogenous group, the student can participate in a larger after-school group with neurotypical peers. Adaptive strategies developed in the homogeneous group can be called on from the individual's growing adaptive repertoire to function more successfully in this community of diverse peers.

Outcome Measures

Improved social participation with the group can be identified by participation in progress of the project and more engagement time with peers. Generalization of improved social participation skills and self-regulation strategies would be observed during the school day or in the community. Improved social participation is also assessed with the Self-Regulation Scale and the Self-Regulation Questionnaire for the teacher.

Formal or informal measurement of relative mastery is carried out and documented. Generalization of social participation skills and satisfaction from the occupational environment is assessed by repeating the Self-Regulation Scale and Self-Regulation Questionnaire results at the end of the group. Peer feedback at the end of the group session with reflection discussion provides the student with feedback from others.

Overall Goal

By addressing issues of social participation for individuals with ASD using preferred interests within an occupational environment group context, occupational therapists are providing the opportunity for addressing the occupational challenge of social participation in a naturalistic context. The occupational adaptation theoretical framework of using preferred

interests or strength-based approaches within a group setting may provide children with ASD with adaptive repertoires they need to improve adaptive functioning for social participation.

Practice Model 12-3: Iraq and Afghanistan Veteran Transition From Active Duty to Civilian Life

Submitted by Christine E. Haines, PhD, OTR

Rationale

- Occupational adaptation provides a lens through which to understand adaptation during times of transition for any population, including veterans who were deployed to Iraq (Operation Iraqi Freedom [OIF]) and Afghanistan (Operation Enduring Freedom [OEF]).
- Occupational adaptation theory recognizes that a veteran's preferred roles are central to the adaptation process and that changes in these roles can lead to occupational dysfunction.
- Occupational adaptation requires consideration of each veteran's motor, process, and interaction skills when planning interventions.
- OIF and OEF service members may benefit from intervention to help restore occupational adaptation from the military context to the civilian context during transition.

Premise

Occupational adaptation is a process that is experienced by every human being (Schkade & Schultz, 1992). Occupation is how people adapt to changing demands, and a person's internal desire for mastery leads to a press for participation in occupation; this desire is the motivational force that leads to adaptation (Schkade & Schultz, 1992). Occupational adaptation is a process that is normative and most pronounced during times of transition (Schkade & McClung, 2001; Schkade & Schultz, 1992). The occupational adaptation process is more important during periods of significant transition because these transitional periods can cause the most disruption in the occupational adaptation process (Schkade & Schultz, 1992). The development of this practice model was based on current research and a qualitative narrative study to describe the transitional process of OIF/OEF veterans through an occupational adaptation lens.

Core Assumptions

- Transition from active duty causes OEF and OIF veterans to experience a loss in role identity and complete change in their occupational environment, resulting in occupational disruption and new occupational challenges.
- OEF/OIF veterans desire mastery in their new civilian roles and environment.
- OEF/OIF veterans come to occupational challenges presented during transition with an adaptation gestalt that might be over- or underactive at any given time during the transition process.
- OEF/OIF veterans leave active duty with ingrained adaptive response modes that were relevant to their roles and environment within the military but may not be relevant to their civilian roles and environment.

Effects of Occupational Dysadaptation

Most veterans transitioning from the military to civilian life feel unprepared for the instability that characterizes the transitional process from the military (Mobbs & Bonanno, 2017) and struggle to generalize adaptive responses to the civilian occupational environment. According to the most recent research, 72% of OEF/OIF veterans experience transitional stress when they leave the military (Mobbs & Bonanno, 2017). This disrupts engagement in occupations of daily living (Kashiwa et al., 2017; Mobbs & Bonanno, 2017; Plach & Sells, 2013) and has been linked to physical and mental health issues, as well as suicidal ideation, with suicide rates among OEF/OIF veterans being 21% higher than their non-veteran peers (Interian et al., 2014; Mobbs & Bonanno, 2017). These consequences can be explained by cyclical experiences of occupational dysadaptation in this population.

Intervention Phases and Strategies

Treatment Approach

Currently, only 60% of returned OEF/OIF veterans seek out health care services with the U.S. Department of Veterans Affairs (Mobbs & Bonanno, 2017). Most will not seek out specific mental health services because of stigmatization but might be found in any other number of treatment settings receiving occupational therapy services (Kashiwa et al, 2017; Mobbs & Bonanno, 2017). Occupational therapists must be aware of the unique needs and challenges faced by this population to provide the best care. The following intervention model can be applied in any setting and is provided as an example based on occupational adaptation principles.

Therapist's Intervention/Process

- Regardless of the reason for referral or treatment setting, the occupational therapist will collect information about the veteran's occupational environments and role expectations.
- The occupational therapist will evaluate the presenting problem and its holistic effect on the veteran's functioning. The presenting problem can be evaluated via traditional methods, but special attention must be directed at all areas of functioning, including psychosocial factors.
- The veteran and the therapist will review the assessment information and jointly determine the relative match between the veteran's role, environmental expectations, and current functioning.
- Therapeutic goals will be developed by the therapist and the veteran. The therapist will determine the plan of care by estimating the veteran's occupational adaptation potential and how to facilitate the potential throughout treatment.

Intervention Methods

- Upon receipt of a referral, determine whether the client is a veteran.
- Perform initial evaluation, rapport building, occupational profile, and current state of functioning.
  - During the initial evaluation, the occupational therapist will build rapport by first gathering background information about the history of their injury and how the injury is affecting their everyday life.
- If the occupational therapist desires a format to guide the interview, the Canadian Occupational Performance Measure might prove helpful, only as a guide. The Canadian Occupational Performance Measure might help guide the occupational therapist in gathering information about how an injury affects the veteran's performance in many different areas of occupation. However, it does not provide specific information about occupational environments or role expectations. Therefore, whether or not the therapist desires a formal guide for the interview portion of the assessment, the occupational therapist must attend carefully to the veteran's occupational environment and role expectations as possible during the assessment interview.

- The occupational therapist then performs objective measurements relevant to the current situation and reviews any recommended protocols with the veteran.
- Together, the occupational therapist and veteran develop a treatment plan focusing on the veteran's specific occupational goals.
- Treatment activities must be relevant to the veteran's functional goals, as well as integrating appropriate adaptive energy, modes, and gestalt during occupational engagement.
- Provide appropriate referrals and additional resources as needed.

While on active duty, service members have high trust in and respect for their medical personnel. This comes from trust required in battle scenarios (Mobbs & Bonanno, 2017). The veteran will likely divulge more information about how occupational environment and role expectations are affecting their daily functioning. The veteran might also begin to talk about issues of loss, grief, stigma, transitional stress, and even suicidal ideation. There are many resources for veterans experiencing transitional problems. The occupational therapist should be aware of some of these resources and understand that many veterans prefer not to engage with these programs. Regardless, the occupational therapist needs to be prepared to address these issues should they arise.

Suggested Typical Phases of Intervention

- Phase I: Assessment and rapport building
- Phase II: Intervention (the phase of intervention will last until all goals are met)
- Phase III: Follow-up and availability

Outcome Measures

Challenges related to transition from the military to civilian life endure for years. Because veteran suicide prevention has been designated a priority by the American Occupational Therapy Association (Kashiwa et al., 2017), it should be expected that veterans will be able to access care throughout their transitional process. Ideally, intervention will last until the veteran has integrated occupational adaptation responses that allow for relative mastery and adaptive functioning in all occupational environments and role expectations.

Overall Goal

The aim of the program is to facilitate ongoing success among veterans transitioning from active duty to civilian life. This process is not necessarily linear and may involve recurring cycles. Ideally, veterans should have access to care from well-informed practitioners whenever stressors interfere with the adaptation process.

Practice Model 12-4: Geriatric Fall Prevention in Inpatient Rehabilitation

Submitted by Brooke King, MSOT, OTR/L

Rationale

More than 1 in 4 adults aged 65 and older fall each year (CDC, 2023a). Falls contribute to serious injury, including fractures, traumatic brain injuries, and death (CDC, 2023a; National Council on Aging, 2020). However, some older adults may be opposed to changes that affect their perceived independence and sense of self. Inpatient rehabilitation is an appropriate venue to address fall prevention because characteristics of the population are correlated with high fall risk, including impairment in balance, gait, strength, sensation, and cognition (Forrest et al., 2012). This transitional period offers an opportunity to integrate evidence-based fall prevention programs that combine consultation, education, and exercise (Elliott & Leland, 2018).

Premise

- Applying a holistic approach to fall prevention makes the topic personally relevant to the individual, increasing the likelihood of carryover.
- The intervention approach targets the individual's desire for mastery.
- Occupational adaptation is holistic, including sensorimotor, cognitive, and psychosocial factors affecting the integration of fall prevention strategies.
- The therapist strategically modulates the occupational environment as an agent of change to facilitate new occupational responses.
- Situating aspects of the intervention in a peer group setting capitalizes on external feedback, which in turn supports the incorporation of adaptive behaviors into one's patterns of behavior.

Core Assumptions

- Fall prevention intervention is critically important to supporting the long-term well-being of older adults.
- Adaptation is stimulated by occupational events. Hospitalization in inpatient rehabilitation typically follows a major injury or health status change, constituting a life event that primes an individual for adaptation to occur.
- A program that facilitates adaptation should take a holistic approach, addressing sensory, mental, and neuromusculoskeletal functioning.

Effects of Occupational Dysadaptation

Occupational dysadaptation takes numerous forms in older adults. For some, it takes the shape of stable patterns, characterized by some rigidity. For example, a maladaptive response to a fall might be to continue navigating the home without a recommended assistive device. Individuals caught in a maladaptive response pattern may continue applying existing modes to solve problems, even as the strategies become less effective because of evolving personal characteristics (such as increasing weakness or deteriorating balance). Making lifestyle changes may clash with the individual's occupational role expectations and self-perception that to be independent means to use no assistive device.

Intervention Phases and Strategies

- Phase I: Initial assessment—evaluation and establishing therapeutic rapport; the therapist identifies the following characteristics related to fall risk and receptivity to change:
  - Sensorimotor traits: Impaired balance, vision, sensation, and motor control correlated with increased fall risk; the occupational therapist assesses and shares findings with the client.
  - Psychosocial traits: Consider the individual's valued roles and responsibilities, perceptions about independence and aging, and prior experiences with therapy and adaptive equipment.
  - Cognitive traits: Memory and attention affect carryover; the cognitive demands of new strategies must match the individual's capabilities.
  - Home environment: Construct a concept of the patient's living situation using a narrative line of questioning to ascertain layout, important features (including stairs, the narrowness of walkways, and bathroom accessibility), and safety characteristics (including security, cleanliness, and general state of repair). This guides intervention toward adaptation that fits with the individual's natural environment.
  - Relative mastery: Establish baseline perception of relative mastery using the Relative Mastery Measurement Scale (RMMS) and the Falls Efficacy Scale (fear of falling) to supplement standard evaluation measures in self-care performance.
- Phase II: Individual treatment—one-on-one interventions supplementing biomechanical remediation strategies with intentional opportunities to generate adaptive responses; at the center of each intervention session is recognition that the client is the agent of change. The therapist and patient complete one-on-one sessions with a focus on scaffolded opportunities to engage in adaptive behavior. The therapist modulates the environment to increase the demand for mastery during occupational performance. Engaging in adaptive response generalization is promoted by involvement with novel challenges in varied environments within the clinic. The therapist focuses on minimizing verbal cuing and physical assist, allowing the client to identify problem areas and generate adaptive responses more independently.
- Phase III: Group sessions—fall prevention group participation; rather than situating education in a culturally unusual social dynamic (a young to middle-aged adult educating an older adult), this practice model embeds a more natural group context so that education is exchanged between peers. The educational component shifted from a pedantic obligation toward an opportunity to engage with peers and to benefit others with one's own knowledge. Each client engages in at least one small group session focused on fall prevention. The therapist facilitates naturalistic interactions between peers structured to stimulate discussion and shared personal narrative related to falls and fall prevention. This authentic, nonthreatening environment allows clients to negotiate new role expectations and explore novel and modified response patterns.
- Phase IV: Reflection, generalization, and discharge—reflection on progress and generalization to the home environment in preparation for discharge

Outcome Measures

As a standard of practice, inpatient rehabilitation clients are evaluated upon admission and re-evaluated in the 3 days leading up to discharge. In this setting, the primary required outcome measure includes assessment of one's independence in activities of daily living, which does include consideration of the individual's safety during task completion. Assessment of self-care tasks offers an occupation-based approach to evaluating adaptive response integration. If relevant, the therapist may assess change in fear of falling with the Falls Efficacy Scale.

The RMMS is an outcome measure specific to occupational adaptation (George et al., 2004). In this model, the scale is useful to gauge the internalization of adaptive behaviors related to safe task completion. Intervention aims to improve an individual's ability to incorporate fall prevention strategies in a satisfactory manner, which is perceived as efficient, effective, and satisfactory to self and others. Using the RMMS as an outcome measure offers objective data to quantify this change.

Overall Goal

Ideally, the outcome is for patients and their therapists to share an improved experience of relative mastery related to fall reduction strategies. Following participation in the intervention, the goal is for a patient to conceptualize fall prevention strategies as effective and efficient, or in other words, worth the required effort. There is an important corollary—to pose the outcome as relative mastery for only the patient participant would be contrived. However, the therapist constitutes an active participant in the client's experience, and as a coevaluator of the fall prevention effectiveness, the therapist's satisfaction is important to consider.

For example, consider the instance when before participation in the fall prevention group, a client endorsed total satisfaction with their home setup and mobility practices even though their therapist noted their physical environment to be characteristic of hoarding and classified their precarious furniture walking as risky to their health. Although the client subjectively experienced relative mastery ("I have never fallen, so I must be doing something right"), the key element of satisfaction also "to others" suggested that, through the therapist's eyes, there was room for improvement. With this individual, the goals of the program were to shift their perception and willingness to sustain change toward a reality more mutually accepted as safe.

Prompts for Further Reflection

Which of these practice models resonates most clearly with your idea of good occupational therapy? Can you envision operationalizing one of these programs in your community? Could you adopt the program but adapt the age group? Or might you be able to use ideas about structure but change the topics or aims? If you could create any program to address a population and problem important to you, how would you start that process?

References

Bauminger, N., & Kasari, C. (2000). Loneliness and friendship in high-functioning children with autism. *Child Development, 71*(2), 447-456.

Benson, B., & Wilcher, M. G. B. (2000). Academic performance among middle school students after exposure to a relaxation response curriculum. *The Journal of Research and Development in Education, 33,* 156-65.

Calm Classroom. (2016, June 15). https://calmclassroom.com/

Centers for Disease Control and Prevention. (2023a, May 12). *Older adult fall prevention: Facts about falls.* https://www.cdc.gov/falls/facts.html

Centers for Disease Control and Prevention. (2023b, March 24). *Prevalence and characteristics of autism spectrum disorder among children aged 8 years: Autism and developmental disabilities monitoring network, 11 sites, United States, 2020.* https://www.cdc.gov/mmwr/volumes/72/ss/ss7202a1.htm?s_cid=ss7202a1_w

Dunst, C. J., Trivette, C. M., & Hamby, D. W. (2012). Effect of interest-based interventions on the social-communicative behavior of young children with autism spectrum disorders. *Center for Early Literacy Learning, 5*(6), 1-10.

Edwards, S., Davis, A. M., Bruce, A., Mousa, H., Lyman, B., Cocjin, J., Dean, K., Ernst, L., Almadhoun, O., & Hyman, P. (2016). Caring for tube-fed children: A review of management, tube weaning, and emotional considerations. *Journal of Parenteral & Enteral Nutrition, 40*(5), 616-622. https://doi.org/10.1177/0148607115577449

Edwards, S., Davis, A. M., Ernst, L., Sitzmann, B., Bruce, A., Keeler, D., Almadhoun, O., Mousa, H., & Hyman, P. (2015). Interdisciplinary strategies for treating oral aversions in children. *Journal of Parenteral and Enteral Nutrition, 39*(8), 899-909.

Elliott, S., & Leland, N. E. (2018). Occupational therapy fall prevention interventions for community-dwelling older adults: A systematic review. *American Journal of Occupational Therapy, 72*(4), 1-11. https://doi.org/10.5014/ajot.2018.030494

Fishbein, M., Benton, K., & Struthers, W. (2016). Mealtime disruption and caregiver stress in referrals to an outpatient feeding clinic. *JPEN Journal of Parenteral & Enteral Nutrition, 40*(5), 636-645. https://doi.org/10.1177/0148607114543832

Forrest, G., Huss, S., Patel, V, Jeffries, J., Myers, D., Barber, C., & Kosier, M. (2012). Falls on an inpatient rehabilitation unit: Risk assessment and prevention. *Rehabilitation Nursing, 37*(2), 56-61. https://doi.org/10.1002/RNJ.00010

George, L. A., Schkade, J. K., & Ishee, J. H. (2004). Content validity of the Relative Mastery Measurement Scale: A measure of occupational adaptation. *OTJR: Occupation, Participation and Health, 24*(3), 92-102. https://doi.org/10.1177/153944920402400303

Interian, A., Kline, A., Janal, M., Glynn, S., & Losonczy, M. (2014). Multiple deployments and combat trauma: Do homefront stressors increase the risk for posttraumatic stress symptoms? *Journal of Traumatic Stress, 27*(1), 90-97.

Kashiwa, A., Sweetman, M. M., & Helgeson, L. (2017). Centennial topics—Occupational therapy and veteran suicide: A call to action. *American Journal of Occupational Therapy, 71*, 7105100010. https://doi.org/10.5014/ajot.2017.023358

Koegel, R., Kim, S., Koegel, L., & Schwartzman, B. (2013). Improving socialization for high school students with ASD by using their preferred interests. *Journal of Autism and Developmental Disorders, 43*, 2121-2134.

Koenig, K. P., & Williams, L. H. (2017). Characterization and utilization of preferred interests: A survey of adults on the autism spectrum. *Occupational Therapy in Mental Health, 33*(2), 129-140.

Law, M. C. (2007). Occupational therapy: A journey driven by curiosity. *AJOT: American Journal of Occupational Therapy, 61*(5), 599-603. https://doi.org/10.5014/ajot.61.5.599

Mobbs, M. C., & Bonanno, G. A. (2017). Beyond war and PTSD: The crucial role of transition stress in the lives of military veterans. *Clinical Psychology Review, 59*, 137-144. https://doi.org/10.1016/j.cpr.2017.11.007

National Council on Aging. (2020). *Falls prevention facts.* https://www.ncoa.org/article/get-the-facts-on-falls-prevention

Pasek, P. B., & Schkade, J. K. (1996). Effects of a skiing experience on adolescents with limb deficiencies: An occupational adaptation perspective. *American Journal of Occupational Therapy, 50*(1), 24-31.

Plach, H. L., & Sells, C. H. (2013). Occupational performance needs of young veterans. *American Journal of Occupational Therapy, 67*, 73-81. https://doi.org/10.5014/ajot.2013.003871

Roux, A., Rast, J., Rava, J., Anderson, K., & Shattuck, P. (2015). *National autism indicators report: Transition into young adulthood.* AJ Drexel Autism Institute.

Rudolph, C. D., & Link, D. T. (2002). Feeding disorders in infants and children. *Pediatric Clinics of North America, 49*(1), 97-112.

Schkade, J. K., & McClung, M. (2001). *Occupational adaptation in practice: Concepts and cases.* Slack Incorporated.

Schkade, J. K., & Schultz, S. (1992). Occupational adaptation: Toward a holistic approach for contemporary practice, part 1. *American Journal of Occupational Therapy, 46*(9), 829-837.

Schkade, J. K., & Schultz, S. (2003). Occupational adaptation. *Perspectives in Human Occupation: Participation in Life*, 181-221.

Schultz, S. (2014). Theory of Occupational Adaptation (pp. 527-540), In B. A. B. Schell, G. Gillen, & M. E. Scaffa (Eds.), *Willard & Spackman's occupational therapy* (12th ed.). Lippincott, Williams & Wilkins.

Schultz, S., & Schkade, J. K. (1992). Occupational adaptation: Toward a holistic approach for contemporary practice, part 2. *The American Journal of Occupational Therapy, 46*(10), 917-925.

Sharp, W. G., Jaquess, D. L., Morton, J. F., & Herzinger, C. V. (2010). Pediatric feeding disorders: A quantitative synthesis of treatment outcomes. *Clinical Child and Family Psychology Review, 13*(4), 348-365.

Sharp, W. G., Volkert, V. M., Scahill, L., McCracken, C. E., & McElhanon, B. (2017). A systematic review and meta-analysis of intensive multidisciplinary intervention for pediatric feeding disorders: How standard is the standard of care? *Journal of Pediatrics, 181*, 116-124.e4. https://doi.org/10.1016/j.jpeds.2016.10.002

Vermeulen, P. (2015). Context blindness in autism spectrum disorder: Not using the forest to see the trees as trees. *Focus on Autism and Other Developmental Disabilities, 30*(3), 182-192.

CHAPTER 13

Setting-Specific Occupational Adaptation Practice Models

*The occupational adaptation practice model
emphasizes the creation of a therapeutic climate,
the use of occupational activity,
and the importance of relative mastery.*
—*Sally Schultz and Janette K. Schkade (1992)*

This chapter offers three examples of practice models that are specific to particular environments: a community-based art studio, a school-based club model, and a hospital-based post-acute rehabilitation program. Although intended for specific locations, the creative occupational therapist will be able to see implications for similar applications in different settings.

Evetts, C. L., & Baxter, M. F. *Cases and Concepts in Occupational Adaptation:
Translating Theory into Action* (pp. 119-129).
DOI: 10.4324/9781003522850-14

Practice Model 13-1: An Art Studio for People With Mental Health Concerns

Submitted by Cynthia Lee Evetts, PhD, OTR, FAOTA

Rationale

Support is needed for community-dwelling people living with mental health concerns. The art studio provides a safe space for self-discovery and self-expression through the creation of visual arts for individuals in the community. Some community members with mental health concerns may be in counseling or therapy, whereas others may not be (due to personal preference or lack of resources). An art studio naturally provides opportunities for doing, being, becoming, and belonging.

Premise

Occupational adaptation is a logical organizing framework for the art studio. Adaptive responses to artistic or creative challenges can be supported, facilitated, or modeled depending on the needs of members. Adaptive responses that lead to a sense of relative mastery in artistic or creative challenges can generalize to occupational challenges in other areas of living a satisfying life in community with others.

Core Assumptions

- Mental health struggles create interruptions in carrying out daily routines that are difficult to predict or control. These interruptions make frequent transitions necessary, and transition creates a higher demand for adaptive processes.
- Seeking feedback from physical and social environments is a natural process in producing visual arts; therefore, an art studio offers opportunities to attend to feedback and experience to improve performance, thereby integrating adaptive responses.
- The ability to experience relative mastery in a desired occupational challenge (like artistic or creative activities) builds adaptive repertoire for use in other challenging occupational activities and roles.

Effects of Occupational Dysadaptation

When people experience distress and lack effective adaptive strategies, they fail to meet both internal and external expectations for fulfilling their occupational roles whether at home, in productive or leisure roles, or in the community attending to instrumental activities of daily living. Failure to meet expectations degrades any sense of relative mastery, which can lead to depressed desires and diminished motivation for engaging in occupational challenges, both required and desired.

Intervention Phases and Strategies

Phase I: Referral and Orientation

- Membership is initiated by referral. Although many mental health providers in the community are made aware of the services and are encouraged to refer clients who may benefit from creative or artistic experiences, self-referral is also accepted.
- Individuals wanting to join the art studio complete a basic questionnaire regarding their primary mental health concerns (diagnosis is not required) and experience with art or art materials.
- The membership coordinator sets an appointment for an orientation (generally outside of studio hours) to go over the code of conduct and get a signed release form and to show the new member what is available in the way of supplies, space, scheduling, and assistance (volunteer artists and mental health mentors who are occupational therapists, art therapists, licensed counselors, and psychologists).
- The new member signs up for a structured session.

Phase II: Structured Opportunities

- It is preferable for new members to first attend structured sessions to:
  - Establish rapport with the volunteer artists and mental health mentors
  - Become familiar with opportunities in the studio
  - Witness the culture and milieu of the art studio

- There are two types of structured opportunities: art classes and therapeutic sessions.
  - Art classes are led by volunteer artists and focus on teaching members specific art-making skills or techniques. Mental health mentors are in attendance for support.
  - Therapeutic sessions revolve around a mindful theme, using art for self-exploration and self-expression with an emphasis on greater self-awareness of adaptive responses to thoughts and emotions related to occupational challenges, interpersonal relationships and/or interactions, and other issues of personal context. Therapeutic sessions are led by mental health mentors (occupational therapists and occupational therapy students). Volunteer artists are in attendance for support. Responsibilities include the following:
    - Planning involves establishing a therapeutic goal for each session.
    - Devise a mindful theme or metaphor to help members grasp and relate to the therapeutic goal.
    - Plan an art-based activity that leans into the theme or metaphor.
    - Ensure that the environmental demands provide a just-right challenge to meet the needs of all members in a session.
      - Because members sign up in advance for a session, the therapist can be ready to grade the challenge for individuals as necessary to promote adaptive responses that will lead to greater relative mastery.
    - The session provides opportunities for members to express their desires.
    - Match desires with demands so that a press for mastery is available to all.
    - Bring awareness to the intentional setting of adaptation gestalt needed to meet a particular challenge. Let members know what to expect. Conduct a centering exercise to calm or alert members as needed to engage in the art making.
    - Facilitate processing by prompting members to share both process and product (encourage and allow but do not require sharing).
      - Provide an opportunity for members to reflect on effective strategies and adaptive responses to challenges and the resulting impact on outcomes.
      - Encourage members to self-assess relative mastery based on efficiency (process), effectiveness (product), and satisfaction to self and others.

Phase III: Open Studio

- During Phase III, members may continue to attend structured sessions while also taking advantage of open studio sessions to:
  - Complete projects begun in structured sessions (repeating successful adaptive responses, being mindful of one's adaptation gestalt)
  - Experiment with new tools, materials, and techniques (using novel tasks and acting as an agent of change)
  - Pursue individual interests (initiating own challenges)
- Mental health mentors continue to support adaptive responses to challenges encountered in the art-making process.
- Volunteer artists facilitate the exploration of materials and techniques and support art-making efforts.

Outcome Measures

Intake and Repeated Measures

- Goal attainment scaling (GAS): The membership application provides an opportunity for indicating what the applicant desires to achieve. GAS(s) are set in collaboration between the member and the mentor. Ideally, a member will have both an artistic goal and a mental health goal, and these will be assessed collaboratively on a monthly or quarterly basis (minimum of four times per year).
- The Depression Anxiety and Stress Scales (DASS-21): The DASS-21 is a 21-item self-report measure with the three subscales indicating the presence of symptoms related to depression, generalized anxiety, and acute stress within the past week. As relative mastery increases, DASS-21 scores are expected to decrease. Measures can be repeated weekly to keep a check on symptom frequency and severity. The frequency of completing the DASS-21 is up to the member.
- The Guide for Occupational Exploration is a semistructured interview yielding a self-report measure of role-related relative mastery and participation.
- Relative mastery: A simple 5-point Likert scale for each component of efficiency, effectiveness, satisfaction to self, and satisfaction of others is available and encouraged at each session, whether structured or open studio.

SAMPLE GOALS

Check the one(s) that you want to work on, or write your own:

ARTISTIC

- ☐ To try out art materials that are new to me
- ☐ To learn new skills with art materials I am familiar with
- ☐ To become comfortable with art materials that I am familiar with
- ☐ To engage with art materials that I am comfortable with
- ☐ To try out art techniques that are new to me
- ☐ To learn new strategies with art techniques that I am familiar with
- ☐ To become comfortable with art techniques that I am familiar with
- ☐ To engage in art techniques that I am comfortable with
- ☐

MENTAL HEALTH

- ☐ To attend sessions on a regular basis
- ☐ To interact with an artist during each session
- ☐ To interact with a mentor during each session
- ☐ To interact with other members during each session
- ☐ To express myself through art
- ☐ To explore my thoughts and/or feelings through art
- ☐ To share my art with others
- ☐ To lower my symptoms of [ ] depression, [ ] anxiety, [ ] stress, [ ] other _____
- ☐ To minimize the impact of [ ] symptoms, [ ] pain, [ ] worries, [ ] strain, [ ] other _____
- ☐ To improve my outlook on life
- ☐ To feel happy/satisfied at the end of each session
- ☐ To respond adaptively when things do not feel right
- ☐ To establish or reinforce a healthy [ ] habit, [ ] hobby, or [ ] routine
- ☐

Guidelines for Volunteers and Mentors to Support Therapeutic Interactions in the Art Studio

Make good use of the following intentional relationship modes of interaction according to Taylor (2008):

- Advocating: speak positively about the art studio, its members, and its mission.
- Collaborating: Work as a team with volunteers and members of the art studio.
- Empathizing: Acknowledge and validate the feelings of others.
- Encouraging: Maintain a positive attitude and promote hope.
- Instructing: Provide clear expectations and direction when needed; do not presume to teach what you do not know.
- Problem solving: Ask questions that lead others to discover solutions.

During all interactions, consider the following components of the recovery model:

- Self-direction: Ask about personal desires, offer choice, and allow deviation.
- Individualized/person centered: Welcome and acknowledge each individual by name.
- Empowerment: Facilitate successful experiences; do not do for, or to, others.
- Holistic: Consider the known and unknown personal context of each individual.
- Nonlinear: All have good and challenging moments; every day is a new day.
- Strengths based: Focus on the positive, build on strengths, and help others see strengths.
- Peer support: Allow members to assist and support each other; promote supportive interactions.
- Respect: Mutual interpersonal respect at all times; respect the studio tools/materials.
- Responsibility: Encourage personal responsibility; take responsibility for own actions.
- Hope: Support positive future orientations.

Consider the following elements of the Pan Occupational Paradigm, an international perspective from occupational science (Hitch & Pepin, 2021):

- Doing: Engaging in occupation (activity) = doing art.
- Being: Reflecting on the meaning of doing = appreciating one's own art, as well as the art of others, identifying as an artist.

- Becoming: Growing and having a future orientation = learning and increasing competence with art materials and techniques.
- Belonging: Putting the doing in context = being a member of the art studio, establishing therapeutic relationships with mentors and volunteers, and making supportive acquaintances and friendships with other members.

Overall Goal

Bottom line: The role of occupational therapy is to use doing (occupation) to facilitate adaptive responses to everyday challenges. Successful experiences in art can generalize to producing adaptive responses in other areas of life.

Practice Model 13-2: Social Participation for Students With Extensive Support Needs: A Friendship Circle

Submitted by Savitha Sundar, MS, OTR/L

Rationale

Designed for students in public school settings, the friendship circle focuses on promoting authentic social inclusion for children with extensive support needs (ESNs) who are often educated in segregated/highly specialized settings. Students with ESNs often lack the skills and opportunities to initiate or engage in social relationships. The overarching goals of this program are social participation, co-occupation, and relative mastery.

Premise

For individuals with ESNs, participation in life's occupations often involves a certain level of co-occupation with caregivers and teachers. Although several students with ESNs may desire social participation and friendships, they may often lack the necessary skills (Müller et al., 2008). If they can collaboratively participate in activities with peers who know and understand them, opportunities are opened for them to participate in several school-related activities they otherwise would miss out on.

Core Assumptions

- When children can become more adaptive, they will become more functional. The experience of mastery is a major motivator for adaptive behaviors.
- Facilitating a therapeutic climate (where the environmental and occupational demands are tailored to facilitate an adaptive response) will help students experience relative mastery, improve self-initiation of tasks, and improve generalization of learned skills/behaviors.
- Occupation is the means for humans to adapt to transition and change in context, and the desire to participate in occupation is the intrinsic motivation for adaptation.
- Adaptation is the change in the functional state of the person due to movement toward relative mastery over occupational challenges.
- For maximal effects on occupational adaptation, the activities, tasks, methods, and techniques of intervention must be centered on occupational activity that promotes satisfaction for the student in the context of school.

Effects of Occupational Dysadaptation

Children with personal system limitations impacting their ability to initiate social interactions are often limited in their experience of social participation. The school environment presents occupational challenges with high demands for social participation that are often beyond their capacity. Within these specialized classrooms, challenges are minimized to match the capacities of the peer group, leaving limited demands to match their desire for social participation. When they become adults, poor understanding of and support for their unique needs in the community leads to large-scale unemployment (occupational deprivation) and isolation when they leave the school system. Individuals with disabilities often desire friendships and greater opportunities to contribute to their community but are more likely to experience profound social isolation (Müller et al., 2008).

A wide range of children with mild disabilities are educated in the general education (gen ed) classroom with few opportunities to experience relative mastery in their main classroom. These students may find the opportunity to be peer mentors a great avenue to display their best selves and experience relative mastery, leading to improved self-confidence and intrinsic motivation. Such an experience is likely to help them to elicit best efforts in other areas as well.

When children grow up with little awareness of the world of disabilities and the role they can play in supporting improved participation for their peers with ESNs in several occupations of life, an attitude of indifference toward individuals with disabilities is likely to reign in their future world. Without real-life social-emotional learning opportunities outside the classroom walls with opportunities to collaborate, initiate, lead, and show empathy, adaptability, and flexibility in real-life situations, children miss out on powerful learning and increased consciousness of the oneness of humankind.

Intervention Approach

- The friendship circle is a programming approach to increase social participation and school success for children with a wide range of abilities and disabilities, although it is primarily focused on those students with ESNs educated in specialized classrooms.
- Members of the education team collaborate to build on students' strengths and address crucial areas of need as they work toward improved relationship development.
- The therapist, as an agent of the environment, facilitates a climate that offers the "just-right challenge" for each student to master and experience success in terms of self-satisfaction, efficiency, and effectiveness.
- Engagement in meaningful occupations and activities is the medium through which participants experience social interactions and relative mastery.
- The program creates hands-on opportunities for students to work collaboratively with peers with different abilities on projects of interest to all. Children learn to be supportive peer role models and mentor peers with social and communication challenges.
- Students from the gen ed population will learn about the world of disabilities and be equipped to act as ambassadors for inclusion within their school community.

Program Phases

The friendship circle meets twice a week for 40 minutes for at least two quarters of the school year.

Phase I: Preparation

- Members of the student's Individualized Educational Plan team will collaboratively design activities and goals according to each student's strengths. These activities will also add value to the school community. Targeted skills will be identified and embedded in the activities by this core team.

- All students with ESNs are in the program.
- After gen ed students have a lesson on disability and an introduction to the program, they are invited to sign up to join the friendship circle.
- The gen ed teacher must approve interested students to participate. The teacher can also recommend and encourage (but not coerce) certain students who may particularly benefit from participation.
- Parents of all children are informed about the program and consent to their child's participation.

Phase II: Participation

- Awareness: Gen ed students learn about the specific disabilities/conditions that peers have, the challenges that come with them, and the gifts they bring to this world through a disability awareness curriculum. Students learn the importance of being compassionate and collaborative. They understand that the purpose of this program is for them to take on a leadership role and assist their peers to have fun in school activities that they may otherwise miss out on.
- Experience: Gen ed students experience entering the world of their peers with disabilities, learning their language (augmentative and alternative communication systems), unique needs (sensory, food choices, etc.), and preferences. They experience how to do an activity together with someone so different in the way they may see/experience the world and yet quite similar to them in other ways.
- Action: They commit to sharing their experiences, thus becoming ambassadors of inclusion in their school community and making the effort to bring in their friends who need them to fully belong to the world of the majority.

Additional Notes on Participation

- A repertoire of activities is available for students to choose from; examples include decorating the school bulletin boards, making holiday ornaments, organizing school dances or other inclusive events, composting school food waste, creating a collage, gardening, putting together goody bags or food bags, shredding, and using shredded paper to make pet beds. The selected activities should be unique to each school's dynamics, needs, and culture.

- The occupational therapist facilitates the selection of appropriate activities that are engaging and meaningful to the participants. Activities must involve active participation, must have an end product that is tangible or intangible, and must be well suited for the particular cohort of students with consideration to financial, temporal, and social factors.
- The expectations for friendship circle members, set by the occupational challenge, include the following:
  - Work on tasks collaboratively with peers (share the load, take turns, communicate with your partner, and have fun).
  - Practice social skills like greeting each other by name, being patient, cooperating, and so on.

Outcome Measures

Outcome measures for students with ESNs are as follows:
- GAS is used to measure progress related to the student's Individualized Educational Plan SMART (specific, measurable, achievable, relevant, and time-bound) goal related to social participation.
- Document demonstration of occupational adaptation as evidenced by the spontaneous response to a peer's social greeting/interaction within the natural context.
- Report self-initiated social interaction in other settings outside the friendship circle as observed by staff.

Outcome measures for gen ed students are as follows:
- Students in gen ed will do monthly repeated measures of self-assessment on the following questions given a sliding scale of 1 to 5 with expression emojis:
  - How much do I know about different disabilities?
  - How comfortable am I working together with someone who cannot talk or understand the world the way I do?
  - When I see a person who needs my help to do well, how likely am I to step up and work together with them?
  - Gen ed students will also rate their level of satisfaction, efficiency, and effectiveness in an identified personal goal on a scale of 1 to 5.

Progress (or lack thereof) is determined by a change in these scores, which will indicate an adjustment in disability awareness, experience, and action.

Overall Goal

The purpose of this program is to create an opportunity for internal transformation in students of all abilities resulting in authentic social inclusion in schools and beyond. Students with ESNs will be more comfortable in the presence of others from having experienced collaborative work with peers, leading to a sense of belonging and improved occupational functioning. Typical peers of children with ESNs are likely to experience relative mastery in the tasks because they are purposefully selected to be fun and engaging in nature. The true challenge is the nurturing of relationships between differently abled peers who may not have previously been responsive to one another. The occupation becomes the medium through which the students experience occupational adaptation.

Practice Model 13-3: Holistic Recovery From Prolonged Hospitalization

Submitted by Michelle S. Scheffler, OTR, MOT

Rationale

Adults who have experienced a prolonged hospitalization because of a medically complex course of events and who are undergoing inpatient rehabilitation as the last part of their hospitalization before returning home are at risk of rehospitalization. Prolonged hospitalization is defined as 3 weeks or greater in an acute care setting. The longer a client is in the hospital (and is effectively institutionalized), the longer the hospital becomes their community, their support system, and their way of daily life. In turn, it becomes more challenging for these clients to begin to transition out of this setting into a home or other community setting. Often the basic occupational functioning and mental health aspects of prolonged hospitalization are not fully addressed with these clients.

Premise

Occupational therapy can help clients who experience prolonged hospitalization achieve relative mastery as they meet new occupational challenges and transition to a nonpatient and goal-directed occupational role. Clients who have difficulty initiating a healthy adaptive response to challenges risk getting stuck in dysadaptive patterns. As a result, it is easy for the client to become withdrawn, dependent on others, and demonstrate poor initiation and ability to adapt overall.

The role of the occupational therapist in facilitating adaptive responses to transition out of a hospital setting into a community setting is vital to clients' success in life and will not be thoroughly addressed by any other health care discipline. Occupational adaptation provides a holistic approach to intervene with clients to truly help them engage in meaningful occupations, achieve adaptive responses to new occupational challenges, assume meaningful occupational roles, and learn to be the agent of change in their lives again.

Core Assumptions

- Humans need to engage in meaningful occupations and adapt to major life circumstances to move forward in life.
  - A person's occupational functioning is changed as a result of an occupational event, and one of the three states of functioning is reinforced: occupational adaptation, homeostasis, or occupational dysadaptation.
  - Occupation provides the means by which humans adapt, and the desire to participate in occupation is the motivation leading to adaptation.
- Occupational deprivation leads to a breakdown in optimal performance and function, as well as a breakdown in the adaptive process when occupational challenges are encountered.
  - All aspects of person systems are present in each adaptive response to occupational challenges.
  - Persons tend to respond to occupational challenges with existing adaptive modes and behaviors, even if these are not appropriate. It is only when the existing modes fail to produce relative mastery that modified or new modes develop.
  - Transitional behaviors offer more promise than hyperstable behaviors because variability brings the possibility of change.
- Humans have an innate desire for mastery that is expressed in meaningful occupational roles. When deprived of meaningful occupations, people may assume a role imposed on them by their environment and/or circumstances.

Effects of Occupational Dysadaptation

Surviving a medically complex and prolonged hospital stay affects the clients' occupational functioning, their adaptive response, and their ability to fulfill their previous occupational roles. Physical, cognitive, and/or psychological changes occur because of the trauma and shock from medical events and complications of illness. Often clients have not had the ability to process what has happened to them and possibly grieve for their former selves. Occupational disruption is certain, and there is a serious risk for occupational deprivation from being in the hospital for a prolonged period. Another risk is loss of role identity due to separation and isolation. The patient role may be fully adopted and difficult to break away from. Persistent dysadaptive modes and behaviors or misuse of adaptive energy results from learned dependence and occupational deprivation. Commonly seen occupational dysadaptation includes paralyzing anxiety surrounding new challenges, depression coupled with poor engagement, withdrawal from basic activities of daily living and previous roles, difficulty conceptualizing the reality of adapting and transitioning to a life outside of the hospital, and difficulty identifying their occupational roles.

Intervention Phases and Strategies

The three overarching objectives are to facilitate (a) the client's generalization of the adaptive response, (b) the development of relative mastery, and (c) the client becoming the agent of change toward any occupational challenge they may meet. The primary tools for intervention are therapeutic rapport and occupation driven by client choice.

Phase I: Initial Assessment

The therapist will meet the client on the first full day in the inpatient rehabilitation unit. The therapist needs to spend time getting to know the client and what is important to them. Collaboratively, the therapist and the client complete an occupational profile to include client-centered goals, building rapport, and setting the stage for the client to become the agent of change in their lives. The goals should also be reasonable and achievable in a realistic time frame. Start with a small goal that the client can engage in and work toward completion on that day to help the client shift out of the patient role and initiate the transition to meaningful roles. Pauses, silence, and open-ended questions are effective in establishing meaningful goals and a therapeutic rapport, allowing the client to think about their responses.

Phase II: Intervention

Include self-care skills or occupational readiness tasks as related to the identified occupational roles. Examples of interventions include the following:

- Activities of daily living and occupational readiness including activities to address sensorimotor challenges, such as transfers, strengthening, endurance, balance, fine motor coordination, and activity tolerance.
- Activities to target cognitive challenges: These must be centered in real-life scenarios. (Paper-and-pencil tasks or simulated scenarios the client may never encounter will not be salient to the clients and do not generalize an adaptive response.) Discussion and feedback after the completion of cognitive tasks also promote the generalization of an adaptive response.
- Interventions to address psychosocial challenges within the context of real-world, everyday scenarios: Interventions can include identifying coping strategies, developing healthy habits and routines that can generalize outside of the hospital setting, identification of and initiation of responsibilities associated with new or pre-existing occupational roles, and guiding the client through a process of self-discovery that results in increased client initiation, self-advocacy, increased feelings of self-worth, and internal measures of success (relative mastery).

Guiding Principles

- Establish a practice of client choice.
  - Whenever possible, give the client a choice of what to work on to target the mutually established goals. This choice sets the stage for how clients will approach their occupations and is key to success. Many clients with prolonged hospitalization are deprived of the opportunity to make choices for themselves as medical professionals do to and for them. It is easy for clients to assume a passive stance as tasks are carried out by team members. Over time, this affects a client's ability to make choices and advocate for themselves.
  - Help the client re-engage in the practice of making choices regarding their care, which will aid in facilitating relative mastery and successful adaptive responses.
  - Consider how the environment can be modified to engage choice making (e.g., location, lighting, sound, time of day, positioning, tools, materials). This can be powerful in bringing clients back to a more familiar sense of self. If clients are struggling, sometimes just engagement in a simple gross motor task and a change of environment, which do not require too much primary energy but more secondary energy, will help the clients take their minds off the situation and allow them to focus more clearly when they complete that simple task.
- Connect client choices to goals, working toward an adaptive response.
  - Design your treatment in such a way that each day the client chooses an activity to work on that is progressive toward their goals. The session should be structured so that the client can see how they are working toward their ultimate goals (e.g., going home, holding a grandchild, working in the yard, walking around the house).
  - Keep these goals at the center of treatment, no matter how simple or challenging they might be. This approach will include dialogue, pauses, silence, open-ended questions, and directing actions and activities back to client goals as each session progresses.
- Client assumes a new or previous role and gains a sense of relative mastery.
  - Watch for a turning point in agency and relative mastery as clients actively come to the treatment sessions with feedback on how activities went outside of therapy, describing challenges that were encountered and met, and thus, demonstrating generalization of an adaptive response.
  - A positive sign of success is observing a client assume a nonpatient role (e.g., mother, worker, grandparent, friend) and gearing their own thought processes, actions, and choices toward carrying out responsibilities associated with that role.

Outcome Measures

Use outcome measures like an Activity Card Sort, Role Checklist, or other self-evaluative assessments, such as a strengths finder. Client measures of relative mastery are encouraged by reflection on the following question: Are you efficient, effective, and satisfying to self and your society? Asking the client each of these questions at regular intervals throughout the treatment will help them to see their progress more from their viewpoint and less from the therapist's, and thus, begin to internalize their adaptation journey.

Overall Goal

The desired change for this client who has experienced prolonged hospitalization is transition toward self-initiated adaptation. We want to see clients who are anxious, depressed, or withdrawn become more engaged, interactive, and advocating for themselves. We want to see an increase in client-initiated decision making. We want to see clients emerge from the role of a patient with learned dependence into a role that is meaningful to them. We want to see a decrease in occupational deprivation and an increase in engagement in meaningful occupations and in role-related behaviors. Most importantly, we want to see an adaptive response that generalizes to novel situations, the client acting as their own agent of change, and the client integrating themselves into a meaningful role upon discharge. The therapist should not simply tell the client, "You don't need me anymore" once the client has generalized the adaptive response; a true indicator of a successful adaptive response will be the client coming to the therapist and stating, "I don't need you anymore."

Do-It-Yourself Mother: A Case of Prolonged Hospitalization

This is the journey and story of a 30-year-old wife, mother, and neonatal intensive care unit nurse. She had an acute onset of Guillain-Barré syndrome, which impacted her ability to speak, swallow, breathe, and physically function. She presented to occupational therapy deconditioned, fatigued, and occupationally deprived after being away from her family and her job. Strengths included her willingness to participate, a strong sense of identity, and the desire to resume previous roles.

Challenges included severe occupational and role deprivation as a result of being in the hospital, physical deconditioning and weakness, and psychosocial deprivation from decreased interaction with her family and loved ones. She was also under a lot of stress due to social factors, such as the unpredictable nature of her husband's military job, an upcoming trip across the state because of his job, and limited childcare options. She missed her children terribly and wondered about the financial implications of not being able to work as she had been used to doing. She was a do-it-yourself mom for her daughters, ages 2 and 4 years.

The occupational therapist and client collaborated to establish goals upon initial assessment. She was initially at minimal assistance for self-care and functional mobility.

Knowing that she would meet self-care goals quickly, the therapist and client structured goals and treatments around the client's ability to return to caring for her two daughters. She also had a remote goal of returning to work. The specific goals included (a) to stand and move around the kitchen and make simple breakfast for her daughters, (b) to play on the floor with her daughters, (c) to change diapers for her 2-year-old daughter, and (d) to get her 4-year-old daughter ready for school in the mornings.

For interventions, the focus was open ended, collaborative, and client driven. Therapy targeted activities of daily living at first to ensure that she could care for herself before attempting to care for others. Sessions included education and compensatory strategies as indicated. The therapist and client then turned their attention to her goals of childcare. The client completed some occupational readiness activities, such as getting in different positions on a therapy mat (all fours, tailor sitting, leaning and reaching, and tall kneeling) to prepare for the multiple positions she would need to assume when chasing down a 2-year-old. The therapist used occupational readiness activities to target balance, core strength, endurance, and safe positioning. Treatment progressed to targeting scenarios she may encounter at home, including adaptations to diaper changing, meal preparation, childcare routines, and general household routines. The therapist and client spent part of one session discussing and educating the client on ways to self-advocate for return-to-work modifications at the appropriate time.

The client went home ready to resume her role as mother and spouse. By the time she left, her confidence level was high; she was engaging throughout the sessions, generalizing techniques and skills she had learned to new situations, and actively collaborating with therapists to problem solve through unique scenarios at home (including environmental barriers and routines for her young children with limited family support).

As the treating therapist, I was sure of the transformation and the generalization of her adaptive response and of her ability to be an agent of change when she sent me a card a few weeks later. In it, she outlined all of the things that she did at home that we had worked on (i.e., making breakfast, caring for herself and her children, completing daily tasks in her role as a wife and mother). The most salient part of the card was that she outlined to me what she had learned from completing those tasks in the home setting. It was her way of saying that she had indeed generalized her adaptive response and that she did not need me anymore—the truest measure of a successful occupational therapy intervention grounded in the theory of occupational adaptation.

Prompts for Further Reflection

Which of these practice models aligns well with your vision of best practice in occupational therapy? Choose a practice model and propose a change to fit the needs in your community. Perhaps you can apply the basic guidelines to a different population or design the intervention for a different practice environment.

References

Hitch, D., & Pepin, G. (2021). Doing, being, becoming and belonging at the heart of occupational therapy: An analysis of theoretical ways of knowing. *Scandinavian Journal of Occupational Therapy, 28*(1), 13-25. https://doi.org/10.1080/11038128.2020.1726454

Müller, E., Schuler, A., & Yates, G. B. (2008). Social challenges and supports from the perspective of individuals with Asperger syndrome and other autism spectrum disabilities. *Autism, 12*(2), 173-109. https://doi.org/10.1177/1362361307086664

Schultz, S., & Schkade, J. K. (1992). Occupational adaptation: Toward a holistic approach for contemporary practice, part 2. *The American Journal of Occupational Therapy, 46*(10), 917-926. https://doi.org/10.5014/ajot.46.10.917

Taylor, R. R. (2008). *The intentional relationship: Occupational therapy and use of self.* F. A. Davis.

Appendix A:
Janette K. Schkade on Adaptive Capacity

The following speech was delivered by Dr. Janette K. Schkade to the class of 2001 during the spring commencement ceremonies at Texas Woman's University. At that time, Dr. Schkade was dean of the Texas Woman's University School of Occupational Therapy.

Your Adaptive Capacity— Don't Leave Home Without It

I want to share some thoughts with you today about something I call adaptive capacity. Obviously, I think it's something important or I wouldn't suggest that you "not leave home without it." So, what do I mean by adaptive capacity? I mean the ability to encounter novel situations (i.e., situations that you haven't encountered before or situations with which you aren't exactly familiar) and find ways to respond to the challenges in those situations—ways that will promote your success and that of others around you.

So, what are the elements of adaptive capacity? There are probably many, but there are three that I want us to think about for a few minutes today. One element is the ability to look around you and find the tools and approaches you need to respond successfully to these unfamiliar events. A second one is to pay attention to what the environment is trying to tell you about how well your response strategies are working. A third one is to recognize your limitations without being limited by them. I'm going to use some personal stories as a way to illustrate what I mean by these three elements.

The first element I'm proposing is to identify and locate the tools you need to respond to unusual challenges. A couple of years ago, I was walking down a favorite road in Arkansas with the man in my life and our dog. After some time, I started to experience a familiar pain in one foot that made it difficult to bear weight on that foot. My very considerate companion suggested that I stay where I was and he would go get the car. So, I sat down on an embankment beside the road to await rescue by my knight in dusty sports utility vehicle. It only took a few moments for me to realize that I would be much more comfortable with back support. I looked behind me and discovered a tree that was of sufficient size to provide that support, so I backed up to the tree. Ah, I thought, this is much better. Then it occurred to me that my offended foot would be more comfortable if I could remove the hiking boot and elevate the foot. Fortunately, there was a rock nearby of sufficient size and relative smoothness to achieve this goal. Now, I thought, I am really set. Wrong! I then discovered that the sun was at such an angle that it was shining directly in my face. I had neither sunglasses nor a cap with a bill. But I did find a twig that had fallen from the red oak tree that was my back support, which had two large leaves, brown, but still attached to the twig. If you know anything about red oak leaves, you know that they have projections that are somewhat like fingers. So, I interlaced the sides of the two leaves and created a relatively solid surface, which I then used to shade my eyes. I felt quite satisfied with this result and complimented myself on this example of adaptive capacity. Now, had another pair of hikers been walking down the road, I'm sure they would have considered me a strange sight. I can just imagine one saying to the other, "Who is that woman with her back to the tree, her foot on a rock, and leaves on her face?" But I thought I had done quite well without the more conventional tools for providing back support, foot elevation, and shade from the bright sun.

The second element of adaptive capacity is to pay attention to what the environment is telling you about the value of your particular strategy. One of our doctoral students in occupational therapy, who is going to graduate today, recently reminded me of an occasion when I was attempting to exit from a parking garage. This particular garage required that the driver place a $1 bill in an electronic bill reader to raise the restricting arm on the exit and allow the driver to get on with life. I prepared myself for this exit by taking out a $1 bill so that I could execute this maneuver speedily and not delay any drivers who might be waiting in line behind me. So, I pulled up to the exit island being careful to get close enough to reach the necessary slot and still not crash into the island itself. I inserted my dollar bill, and the device rejected my dollar and returned it to me. I thought perhaps it is one of those readers that require the bill to have a certain orientation, so I rotated it 180 degrees and reinserted it. Once more the bill was returned to me. I was beginning to think someone had given me a counterfeit bill. I turned the bill over and tried again, once more without success. I rotated it 180 degrees with the same result. By now, cars are starting to line up behind me. Being convinced that my bill was bogus, I rifled around in my purse for my wallet, and fortunately, I had one more dollar bill available. I inserted the new bill into the slot, and this bill was also returned to me. I noticed in my rearview mirror that the woman in the car directly behind me had opened her door and was walking toward me. There was no parking garage rage here. No one in line was honking a horn or shouting obscenities. The now ambulatory driver from behind me came to my window and said very matter-of-factly, "The arm is up." This was one of those freebie days that you always long for when you can exit without paying.

Evetts, C. L., & Baxter, M. F. *Cases and Concepts in Occupational Adaptation: Translating Theory into Action* (pp. 131-132).
DOI: 10.4324/9781003522850

My previous experience in this parking garage had led me to believe that without a successful execution of the "feed the electronic slot maneuver," I would be unable to exit for lack of the proper currency. The trouble was that I had not been paying attention to what the environment was telling me. I had decided on one strategy that had worked for me before in this very garage. But instead of taking the failure as an environmental cue to look around me and consider other possibilities, I persevered with a previously successful but now unsuccessful, and as it turned out, unnecessary strategy. My error was in focusing on where I had been instead of where I was going.

So, a second element of adaptive capacity is to pay attention to what the environment is telling you about your strategy. If it isn't working, you need to abandon it and look for other alternatives.

A third element is to be aware of your limitations without being limited by them. This may sound like a contradiction in terms, but it isn't really. I get concerned when I hear people say that "You can be anything you want to be." You see, I don't think that's exactly true. When I was a teenager, I decided that I wanted to grow up to be tall, slender, and demure. Well, it didn't work out that way. Instead, you see before you someone who is rather short, a bit dumpy, and a tad rowdy. And never, in my most youthful and supple years, could I have hurled myself into space to do tumbling runs as I have seen gymnasts do. Nor could I have ever painted a picture that someone would purchase and display on the walls of the Kimball Art Museum. I was never in danger of being invited to perform a solo concert at Carnegie Hall to standing room–only crowds and thunderous applause.

Despite my own limitations, I have had some successes that have given me great joy as I think back on my career. I have been blessed to teach wonderful occupational therapy students who led me to believe that my ideas were of value. Some of those students have worked with me over the years to develop and refine those ideas. I have had the honor to collaborate with an outstanding occupational therapy faculty whose adaptive capacity I have challenged in recent years beyond any bounds they might have imagined, and they have responded magnificently. I have had the privilege of participating in many deliberations with fellow deans in mutual pursuit of an educational environment characterized by both excellence and caring. Despite my limitations, these opportunities have been mine to experience.

Each discipline represented in this graduating group today has encountered its own set of adaptive challenges. Occupational therapy, where my heart lives, is in the business of adaptation. Our therapeutic function is to have an impact on the adaptive capacity of our patients. Why? So that those patients, in whose lives we intervene, can occupy their time in ways and in manners that are personally meaningful to them in spite of illness, trauma, or loss.

When each of you emerges from this ceremony today, you will embark on your own professional journey. You must decide what you will take with you and how you will pack your professional tools and treasures for the journey ahead. Of course, you will pack your knowledge base. This is the foundation within which you think about what you do and the ways you can extend and expand your practice. Of course, you will pack your professionalism. Along with your knowledge base, it gives you credibility and the opportunity to influence and contribute to the larger professional world around you. I trust that you will also pack your adaptive capacity. Pack it where it is easily accessible. Take it out and exercise it so it gets stronger, more creative, and more versatile. The stronger it is, the more it can withstand the rigors and uncertainties of the luggage handling processes of professional life.

I have a friend named Jane. When you ask her how things are going at work, she responds with a characteristic comment. "Oh," she says, "I'm just struggling from ditch to ditch." What she's referring to are the ups and downs that will invariably confront you as you go about your professional lives. Although you can't avoid the ups and downs, you do have a choice about whether you carry with you a shovel or a ladder. With the shovel, you can dig yourself in deeper. With the ladder, you have a way to climb out. I would suggest that the ladder is your adaptive capacity.

So, the three ideas that I hope you will take with [you] about your adaptive capacity are:

1. Remember to look around you and find the tools that can be useful in helping you to deal with unexpected situations and challenges. This is particularly important when standard approaches don't seem to be available.

2. Pay attention to what the environment is telling you about the success or failure of your strategies. Change them if you need to.

3. Recognize your limitations but don't be limited by them. The world is filled with marvelous opportunities by which you can fulfill your dreams and desires.

That's your adaptive capacity—don't leave home without it!

—*Janette K. Schkade, May 12, 2001*

Appendix B:
Worksheet Answer Keys

The following pages include answer keys to worksheets presented in this book.

Evetts, C. L., & Baxter, M. F. *Cases and Concepts in Occupational Adaptation: Translating Theory into Action* (pp. 133-137).
DOI: 10.4324/9781003522850

CASE 3-3 WORKSHEET
The Video Gamer Challenge

Potential responses include but are not limited to what is presented in gray.

List the definitions and descriptions of the words, diagnoses, abbreviations, or processes that you investigated.

Words/phrases: postnatally, pulmonary atresia, pulmonary arch, bilateral superior vena cava draining to coronary sinus, pulmonary angioplasty, heart catheterization, disconjugate gaze, alternate patching of his eyes, chest tube, pulse-oximeter, g-tube, telemetry leads, sternal incision

Abbreviations: RV-PA, ASD, ADLs

Diagnoses: Tetralogy of Fallot

Bonus: Which therapies did Charlie most likely receive before this hospitalization?

The American Occupational Therapy Association offers a specialty certification in Feeding, Eating, and Swallowing, reinforcing the understanding that this is not an entry-level area of practice. Clinical evaluation of feeding and swallowing is also an area of practice for speech therapists.

Describe Charlie's typical and immediate contexts; include both personal and environmental factors.

- Be sure to distinguish between the facts you know and the assumptions you may have made based on what you know.

TYPICAL Context: Facts (F)/Assumptions (A)	IMMEDIATE Context: Facts (F)/Assumptions (A)
Only child living at home with his mom (F) and dad (A), private room (A) with parent/s nearby (A), access to outdoors (A)	Semiprivate (A) room in the cardiovascular intensive care unit (F) with hospital bed with rails, bedside chair, window
Homeschooled (F) with decreased interaction with same-age peers (A) or authority figures other than mom (A)	Limited interaction with anyone except hospital staff (A)
Street clothes—jeans, t-shirts, sweats, shoes (A)	Hospital gown, gripper socks, monitors with lines, tubes, stitches (F)
Video games (F)	TV with preselected (limited) channels (A), game system (F)

- How can you confirm your suspicions? In other words, what is necessary to turn assumptions into the knowledge of facts? Talk to Charlie. Assumptions are questions that need to be answered to have an accurate picture of the client's actual context.

Speculate on possible reasons why Charlie may have refused activities of daily living during his first meeting with the occupational therapist. Consider both internal and external expectations related to Charlie's occupational role(s).

He had been told to stay put and not get out of bed or do anything unless the nurse was there.

He did not know the occupational therapist and was embarrassed to do ADLs in front of her.

He was afraid it might hurt or set his recovery back.

He was testing his ability to assert autonomy with the occupational therapist.

He had already done ADLs that day.

He was tired.

In this scenario, what was the environmental demand for Charlie?

Listen to the doctors and nurses and do what they say.

Restrict movement to avoid pulling out lines, leads, and tubes.

Take medicine, submit to medical procedures.

What was Charlie's desire?

To be a kid, go home, and play video games.

What provided press for mastery via a just-right occupational challenge?

Opportunity to play a video game also set the stage for getting out of bed, getting dressed, and toileting; ambulating, standing and sitting tolerance; upper extremity endurance with minimal resistance.

Bonus: Which of Charlie's favorite games would you recommend he engage in and why?

Is Minecraft good for kids? Yes, Minecraft is educational because it enhances creativity, problem solving, self-direction, collaboration, and other life skills. In the classroom, Minecraft complements reading, writing, math, and even history learnings. Both fun and educational, Minecraft is easily on our list of best video games for kids. (iD Tech. [2016, June 7]. Is Minecraft good for kids? 3 big educational benefits [Blog]. *iD Tech*.)

Fortnite is harmful for kids. First of all, it can be addictive. Sure, it doesn't show blood, but players still kill each other, and that's too intense for kids. The game is free, but it pushes players to spend money to buy extras, like dance moves for the characters. (Storyworks 3. [2018, September 3]. Is Fortnite OK for kids? *Scholastic*.)

A DEEPER DIVE WORKSHEET

The Vacationer

Potential responses include but are not limited to what is presented in gray.

Read Carandang, K., & Pyatak, E. A. (2018). Analyzing occupational challenges through the lens of body and biography. *Journal of Occupational Science, 25*(2), 161-173. https://doi.org/10.1080/14427591.2018.1446353.

Create a list of definitions/descriptions of the words, diagnoses, abbreviations, or processes that you need to understand better.

Diagnoses: Type 1 diabetes, blood glucose levels, hemoglobin A1C

Abbreviations: DMV

Describe Sadie's typical and immediate contexts; include both personal and environmental factors.

• Be sure to distinguish between what you know and the assumptions you may have made based on what you know.

TYPICAL (HOME) Context: Facts (F)/Assumptions (A)	IMMEDIATE (COLLEGE) Context: Facts (F)/Assumptions (A)
No alcohol (F)	Frequent outings to bars/pubs (F)
Mom provides instructions for self-care (F)	Autonomy in decision making (F)
Reinforced routines and habits (F)	Freedom to delay or abandon routines (F)
Diabetes camp camper (F)	Diabetes camp counselor (F)

Speculate on possible reasons why Sadie may have neglected her health-maintenance role. Consider both internal and external expectations related to Sadie's occupational role(s).

Conflicting external demands, social (friends) vs. medical (doctors).

Medical criteria targets that move so efforts are "never good enough".

Wanting to live a "normal" life without the added responsibilities of attending to diabetes.

Not wanting to appear dependent on her condition among her friends.

In this scenario, what was the environment demanding of Sadie?

College classes require that you show up on time and stay attentive during class, do assignments and turn them in on time.

Friends may demand spontaneous change of plans without regard to lifestyles outside of their own experience.

How are the concepts of body state and biographical moment congruent or discordant with explanations of the occupational adaptation process (specifically internal and external role expectations)?

The idea of body state is consistent with OTPF description of body functions, which influence internal expectations (if we heed our body) and external expectations of physicians or other care providers who are responding to the body-state/function …

The idea of a biographical moment is supported by temporal context, personal factors (such as behavioral patterns, identity, lifestyle, and health conditions) and influenced by values, beliefs, and spirituality (client factors).

Bonus: What would you recommend for Sadie and why?

I would try to tap into Sadie's desire for mastery and help her realize that attending to her body's needs will greatly influence how well she will be able to achieve her goals, in the immediate circumstances and in the long run toward the future she envisions.

CASE 8-1 WORKSHEET

The Lineman

Potential responses are provided in gray, yet the representative responses should not be presumed to be fully reflective nor fully inclusive for all children.

Name the occupation in context, and then list all aspects of the occupational environment. Consider how each environmental aspect presents expectations and feedback and how the occupational response may change aspects of the occupational environment.

Occupation: Peewee football lineman, plays on a team with other similarly aged peers with goals to have fun, please parents, and make friends.

Environment	Expectation	Feedback	Adaptive Response	Incorporation
Physical/Nonhuman				
Outdoor grassy field	Soft surface for running/falling	Grass tickles skin or is itchy, stains cloths/skin	Jump up quick when you go down	Over time, the grass is worn down/compressed
Uniform	Identify players	Cues to identify self and others	Wear the uniform	Spectators recognize belonging for those in uniform
Safety gear	Protect against injury	Is hot, heavy, proprioceptive input	Add sweatband/skull cap to keep sweat off face	Becomes part of the uniform
Prolate spheroid-shaped ball	Spirals when thrown	Ball is hard, hurts if caught wrong	Linebackers are defensive; job is to prevent others passing/catching the ball	Peewee balls are softer, smaller; defensive players are not expected to catch passes
Social				
22 kids per team	Cooperate, share, support/protect, be friendly	Smiles, inclusion	Learn to reciprocate friendly gestures	Cohesive team
2 to 4 coaches	Follow directions, remember the rules, show up, and try hard	Encouragement, direction and correction, praise	Listen for directions, watch successful peers, risk trying	Coordinated team efforts
Parents on the sidelines	Be safe, have fun, play to win	Cheer, shout encouragement	Continue playing, help the team	Team success/cohesiveness
Cultural				
Football is aggressive	Play hard, run fast, push hard	Getting pushed back	Sustain push for desired sensory input	Praise/cheers for effective blocking
Aggressions are restricted to sanctioned plays	Be careful not to hurt self or others, learn to block effectively	Trust safety gear, have empathy for others	Block effectively, regulate impulses, save strength and effort for plays	Team with a strong defense

A DEEPER DIVE WORKSHEET

Therapeutic Ingredients

*A sample of on-target responses are provided in gray. You may have worded things differently
to create a sound argument grounded in occupational adaptation concepts.*

For each of the recommended therapeutic ingredients, write a statement that links the intervention strategy to the theory of occupational adaptation and answers the following question: "Why is this important?"

THERAPEUTIC INGREDIENT	WHY? (LINK TO THEORY)
Intentionally provide opportunities to select, plan, and execute meaningful activity and evaluate task performance	The client is the agent of change and the expert on their own life and desires for mastery. Conscious self-assessment of relative mastery will enhance the chances of adaptive response integration to build adaptive repertoire.
Intentionally provide opportunities to create tangible products or intangible but recognizable outcomes	Assessment of relative mastery is related to an outcome of an occupational challenge.
Intentionally provide opportunities to engage in graded, just-right occupational challenges	Success results in feelings of relative mastery that spark additional desires for mastery. This is a strength-based approach to building adaptive capacity.
Intentionally provide opportunities to receive direct or indirect verbal or physical assistance only as necessary	Intervening too soon may rob the client of true feelings of relative mastery—"I did it myself." Allowing deep failure may thwart future attempts and desires.
Intentionally provide opportunities to receive objective, nonjudgmental feedback	Honest, constructive feedback helps the client achieve useful self-appraisal. Withholding judgment (like/dislike) allows the client to be the judge; ultimately, their own sense of relative mastery matters most.
Intentionally provide opportunities to participate in novel tasks or contexts	A sign of improved occupational adaptation is generalization to novel tasks and situations.
Intentionally provide opportunities to engage in a positive social environment	Social interaction is part of environmental feedback. A positive environment is more conducive to growth and adaptive behavior.
Intentionally provide opportunities to experience self in an occupational role that is personally satisfying	Even in group settings, each client ought to be able to link therapeutic tasks to their individually selected meaningful occupational roles.

Financial Disclosures

Alondra Ammon reported no financial or proprietary interest in the materials presented herein.

Lindsay Ballew reported no financial or proprietary interest in the materials presented herein.

Dr. Mary Frances Baxter reported no financial or proprietary interest in the materials presented herein.

Gail Blom reported no financial or proprietary interest in the materials presented herein.

Dr. Jessica Dolecheck reported no financial or proprietary interest in the materials presented herein.

Dr. Cynthia Lee Evetts reported no financial or proprietary interest in the materials presented herein.

Dr. Christine E. Haines reported no financial or proprietary interest in the materials presented herein.

Catherine Evich Johnson has not disclosed any financial or proprietary interest in the materials presented herein.

Jessica Johnson reported no financial or proprietary interest in the materials presented herein.

Dr. Kristin Bray Jones reported no financial or proprietary interest in the materials presented herein.

Dr. Kyle Karen reported no financial or proprietary interest in the materials presented herein.

Brooke King reported no financial or proprietary interest in the materials presented herein.

Joanna Lipoma has not disclosed any financial or proprietary interest in the materials presented herein.

Dr. Christene Mass reported no financial or proprietary interest in the materials presented herein.

Kimberly Norton has not disclosed any financial or proprietary interest in the materials presented herein.

Emily M. Rich reported no financial or proprietary interest in the materials presented herein.

Dr. Stefanie Casey Rogers reported no financial or proprietary interest in the materials presented herein.

Dr. Teri K. Rupp reported no financial or proprietary interest in the materials presented herein.

Dr. Sarah Rupp-Blanchard reported no financial or proprietary interest in the materials presented herein.

Michelle S. Scheffler reported no financial or proprietary interest in the materials presented herein.

Stephanie Springfield has not disclosed any financial or proprietary interest in the materials presented herein.

Dr. Anne Sullivan reported no financial or proprietary interest in the materials presented herein.

Savitha Sundar reported no financial or proprietary interest in the materials presented herein.

Nanette Tabani has not disclosed any financial or proprietary interest in the materials presented herein.

Dr. Orley A. Templeton reported no financial or proprietary interest in the materials presented herein.

Jennifer K. Whittaker reported no financial or proprietary interest in the materials presented herein.

Story/Case Index

Index